Working with Families in Early Intervention

Infants & Young Children Series

Edited by

James A. Blackman, MD, MPH

Professor of Pediatrics
Director of Research
Kluge Children's Rehabilitation Center and Research Institute
Department of Pediatrics
University of Virginia
Charlottesville, Virginia

AN ASPEN PUBLICATION®
Aspen Publishers, Inc.
Gaithersburg, Maryland
1995

Library of Congress Cataloging-in-Publication Data

Working with families in early intervention/
edited by James A. Blackman.
p. cm.
A collection of articles from the journal
Infants and young children.
Includes bibliographical references and index.
ISBN 0-8342-0646-3
1. Handicapped children—Rehabilitation.
2. Family Services. I. Blackman, James A.
II. Infants and young children.
[DNLM: 1. Family Therapy—collected works.
2. Family—collected works.
3. Maternal Health Services—collected works.
4. Child Welfare—collected works.
WM 430.5F2 W926 1995]
RJ138.W67 1995
362.1'9892—dc20
DNLM/DLC
for Library of Congress
94-38450
CIP

Editorial Resources: Amy Myers-Payne

Library of Congress Catalog Card Number: 94-38450
ISBN: 0-8342-0646-3
Series ISBN: 0-8342-0652-8

Printed in the United States of America

1 2 3 4 5

Table of Contents

Preface

The family is a subject on which everyone is expert. We have all been a part of some kind of family at some time. Perhaps the feelings we draw from that experience are happy and warm or possibly sad and unpleasant; yet, when we are not part of some kind of family, even temporarily, we feel empty, lonely, and unsupported. Conversely, a strong family connection gives us energy, confidence, and a sense of well-being.

With such universal expertise, why has the recent emphasis on family-centered care seemed so novel and required such a reordering of how we behave professionally? Somehow what we did professionally and what we all needed so much in our personal lives did not connect. But it connects now and we will never be able to return to our autocratic way of treating clients or patients, especially when health and welfare reform remove financial dependency on insensitive government and private service delivery agents.

Our society is finally rediscovering that its disintegration is likely if we let the concept of family continue its slide toward neglect. Several recent legislative actions, such as the Family Leave and Family Preservation Acts, finally acknowledge that the critical unit of society is not the individual or a nation, but the family. Developing a national family support policy, and perhaps a bureau to coordinate activities in support of this policy, should be a top political priority. The early intervention law, Public Law 99-457 (IDEA), has been an important impetus in this country for renewed interest in strengthening, if not saving, the family.

This volume is replete with ideas about how to support families in a variety of circumstances. Family-centered service is a philosophical tenet we all must internalize in early intervention; but the practical application of this philosophy, once embraced, requires thought, ingenuity, experimentation, and continuing re-evaluation. Making early intervention family-centered will not only enhance the likelihood of success, it will promote the importance of the family in all spheres of our society.

James A. Blackman, MD, MPH
Editor

A flexible and functional approach to developing individualized family support plans

Angela G. Deal, MSW
Coordinator, Child and Family Services

Carl J. Dunst, PhD
Director

Carol M. Trivette, MA
Research Associate
Family, Infant and Preschool Program
Western Carolina Center
Morganton, North Carolina

CONSTRUCTING any type of building begins with some idea of what the structure will look like and what purpose it will serve. Architects take such ideas and use them to design and draw plans for the building. These architectural drawings are the blueprints that builders depend on for erecting the structure. Without the benefit of blueprints, the completed building may not be or do what the originator had in mind.

Building family support programs also begins with some idea of what the programs ought to look like and what purposes they should serve.[1–4] The architects of these programs formulate plans that guide program development and implementation. The plans serve as blueprints for building support systems and mobilizing community resources that will produce intended outcomes. Without the benefit of blueprints, program building efforts may not have anticipated impacts.

The passage and enactment of Public Law 99-457 (Education of the Handicapped Act Amendments of 1986) marked entry into a new era for those interested in building support programs for handicapped children and their families. Part H of the law established a discretionary early intervention program designed to meet the special needs of handicapped infants and toddlers and their families. The cornerstone of the Part H provisions is the Individualized Family Support Plan (IFSP). The IFSP is the blueprint for guiding resource mobilization designed to meet child and family needs. Congress intended that families themselves be the architects of the IFSP[5] and that early-intervention practitioners assist families in acquiring the knowledge and skills necessary to build support systems that strengthen family functioning.[1,4]

The approach to developing and implementing IFSPs described in this article is based on principles and guidelines for practice designed to support and strengthen

The development of the methods and procedures described in this article was supported, in part, by grants from the U.S. Department of Health and Human Services (#0090DD0113 and #90CA124602), U.S. Department of Education (#G008530078), and the North Carolina Children's Trust Fund (#C9514 and #C1130). Special thanks to Laura Gentry, Ginna Wheatley, Karen Holbert, Nancy Watts, Nancy Gordon, Donald Kantner, Debbie Kantner, Leesa Schoeberle, Renne Harrison, Gail Harrison, Lola Harrison, Tim Truemper, Lisa Shetts, Michelle Davis, Benny Hudgins, and Cora Hudgins for assistance in field testing the version of the IFSP described in this article.

Inf Young Children 1989; 1(4): 32–43

family functioning.[1] It has been developed within the context of a needs-based family systems model of assessment and intervention.[4] The process for developing IFSPs is designed to be both flexible and functional in order to be continually responsible to the concerns and needs expressed by families. The format for writing IFSPs is also flexible and functional to ensure that the plan reflects the transactions that occur between the members of the family's social network designed to mobilize resources to meet needs.

A FAMILY SYSTEMS ASSESSMENT AND INTERVENTION MODEL

The family systems model and the IFSP process are based on a set of conceptual underpinnings and principles for practice that guide resource mobilization to meet family needs. This model is briefly described to place the approach to developing IFSPs in proper perspective.

Conceptual bases

The implementation of the assessment and intervention model is guided by a number of beliefs that emphasize a proactive, highly responsive approach to working with families. First, major emphasis is placed on both enabling and empowering families.[6–10] *Enabling* families means creating opportunities for family members to become more competent and self-sustaining with respect to their abilities to mobilize their social networks to get needs met and attain desired goals.[1] For example, assisting families in meeting needs provides experiences and opportunities for acquiring skills that will be useful as part of future efforts to obtain resources to meet new needs and challenges. *Empowering* families means carrying out interventions in a manner in which family members acquire a sense of control over their own developmental course as a result of their efforts to meet needs.[7,11,12] That is, as families experience success in accessing resources, their confidence in their own abilities to handle future challenges is greatly enhanced.

Second, major emphasis is placed on strengthening both families and their natural support networks without either usurping their decision-making power or supplanting their personal social support networks with professional services.[1] Strengthening families means supporting and building on the things the family already does well as a basis for promoting and encouraging the mobilization of resources among the family's personal social network members.[13]

Third, major emphasis is placed on enhancing families' acquisition of a wide variety of competencies that permit them to become capable of meeting needs through mobilization of their support networks. Enhancing the acquisition of competencies means providing families with the information and skills necessary for them to become more self-sustaining and thus better able to solve problems and meet needs, which in turn is likely to have positive influences in other areas of family functioning.[6,9,10,14–16] Enabling, empowering, and strengthening families constitute the major goals of the assessment and intervention process.

Principles for practice

The assessment and intervention model is based on four principles derived from a converging body of empirical and clinical evidence[4] regarding the essential components and elements of effective helping.[7,9,10]

Principle 1: Intervention efforts should be based on family-identified needs and aspirations in order to have the greatest positive influences on child, parent, and family functioning. This principle is based on evidence that establishes a functional relationship between needs (desires, aspirations, personal projects) and a number of aspects of family functioning, including well-being and adherence to professionally prescribed regimens.[17] One theme that has surfaced repeatedly as part of the present authors' research and clinical experience is that interventions implemented in response to family-identified needs are more likely to have second- and higher-order influences[18] on a number of aspects of parent, child, and family functioning.[6,15,19]

Principle 2: Existing family strengths and capabilities (family functioning style) should be built on as a basis for promoting the family's ability to mobilize resources in order to enhance successful efforts toward meeting needs. The second principle is derived from evidence regarding the capabilities that constitute family strengths, and how family functioning style affects the ability to deal effectively with normative and nonnormative life events and promotes growth in all family members.[4] The authors' work with families has demonstrated that knowledge of family strengths and capabilities provides the basis for building on the things a family already does well, and that doing so is more likely to result in the family's investment of time and energy to mobilize resources.

Principle 3: The family's personal social network should be strengthened, and use of untapped sources of aid and assistance should be promoted, in order to ensure the availability and adequacy of resources for meeting needs. The third principle is based on evidence that shows that the most powerful benefits of support are realized if aid and assistance come primarily from informal sources.[16,19] Experience tells the present authors that many early-intervention practitioners fail to consider the full range of social support options available to families. Consequently, there is a tendency to overprofessionalize services to handicapped children and their parents. A rule of thumb in mobilizing resources to meet needs is never to provide aid or assistance that the family can obtain from sources of support closer to the family unit.

Principle 4: Helping behaviors should be employed that promote the family's acquisition and use of competencies and skills necessary to mobilize and secure resources in order to enhance the family's ability to become more self-sustaining with respect to meeting their needs. The ability to attain this goal is guided by a proactive approach to working with families, a shift and expansion in the roles professionals employ in working with families, and a set of guidelines that has both enabling and empowering consequences when used to structure intervention practices.[4] This principle is derived from evidence that demonstrates that different ways of helping have differential effects on a person's ability to become more self-sustaining.[9,10] The authors' research and clinical experiences with mobilizing resources to meet family needs has demonstrated that it is not just a matter of whether needs are met but rather the manner in which mobilization of resources and support occurs that is a major determinant of enabling and empowering families.[6,9,10] To be both enabling and empowering in a way that promotes a family's capabilities and competencies, the family must be actively involved in the process of identifying and mobilizing resources, and the interventionist must derive personal and intrinsic gratification and enjoyment from seeing others become more capable and competent.[20]

Figure 1 graphically shows the four operational components of the family systems assessment and intervention model and relationships among the components. Family needs and aspirations, family strengths and capabilities (family functioning style), and social support and resources are seen as separate but interdependent elements of the assessment and intervention process. The help-giving behaviors used by professionals are seen as the ways in which families are enabled and empowered to acquire and use competencies to procure support and mobilize resources for meeting needs.

The process of enabling and empowering families can be thought of as a system of interlocking gears (needs and aspirations, family strengths and capabilities, support and resources) that must be properly aligned if motion and energy are to be passed from one gear to another. Each gear in the system serves a specific function and, when properly adjusted, generates energy and power that make the parts of the whole contribute to optimal efficiency.

The dynamic processes that make up the family system can be likened to those on a touring bike where, at any given time, one gear plays a more important role, but it is still the particular alignment among all gears that generates momentum, speed, energy, and power. The latter set of characteristics is primarily influenced by two factors: the terrain (developmental course) that is being traversed by the family and the capabilities necessary for the family to drive the system forward in a positive direction.

Conceptualizing the relationship among needs and aspirations, strengths and capabilities, and resources and support as an interlocking set of gears that forms a system generating energy and power requires a shift in the ways professionals have typically worked with families. The goal is not for the professional to take

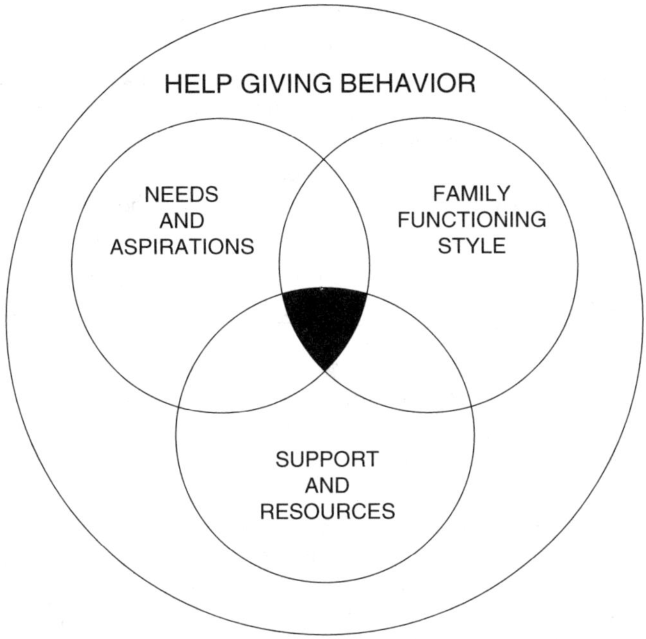

Fig 1. The four major components of the family systems assessment and intervention model.

---

control of the system and define the family's developmental course. Rather, the goal becomes one of promoting the family's ability to negotiate alignment of the gears comprising the system in a way that makes the system operate as efficiently as possible.

WRITING FLEXIBLE AND FUNCTIONAL IFSPs

The family systems assessment and intervention model described above has been used to develop both a process and format for developing and writing IFSPs. The process is intended to be continually responsive to the changing needs of children and families. The format for developing and implementing IFSPs is both flexible and functional, and it is designed as a blueprint for capturing the details of what is accomplished as part of mobilizing resources to meet family needs.

As part of their efforts to help families identify their needs and mobilize resources for meeting needs, the present authors have found it useful to distinguish between static and fluid intervention plans as a basis for proposing a more flexible and functional approach for developing and implementing plans to meet family-level needs. A static plan is one that does not permit, or at least discourages, frequent changes and modifications once goals, methods, and outcomes have been specified. In contrast, a fluid plan is one that not only permits but encourages frequent modifications as a result of the changes that occur in a family, including the situations that influence family behavior and any other conditions that affect child and family behavior. A fluid plan is one that is responsive to the changing needs of families and therefore is both flexible and functional.

Guiding principles

The process of developing IFSPs is guided by a number of principles that enable, empower, support, and strengthen family functioning. The principles are based on conceptual and pragmatic considerations described elsewhere.[1,14,21]

First, development of the IFSP is done within the context of collaboration and partnerships between the family and early-intervention practitioner. *Collaboration* means cooperation among people. *Partnership* means an association among people and the pooling of resources in pursuit of some common or joint interest. Collaborative and partnership arrangements between the family and early-intervention practitioner increase the likelihood that, as a team, mobilization of resources will occur in a manner that achieves stated intentions because of shared responsibility.[22,23]

Second, any and all information included in the IFSP is done so with the explicit permission and authorization of the family. The content of the IFSP need not be intrusive or violate confidentiality if the family, as architect of the IFSP, retains final decision-making power with respect to its full content. This principle recognizes the family's rightful role to decide what is important for the family unit and individual family members, and that the family alone bears the responsibility for deciding their developmental course to the extent that the well-being and rights of all family members are protected. The early-intervention practitioner helps the family make informed decisions by providing whatever information, aid, and assistance necessary for the family to choose what they consider is in their best interest.[23]

Third, the development and revision of the IFSP should be responsive to the broad-based needs of families, although no early-intervention practitioner or program should be expected to offer support to meet all family needs. This principle includes two important interrelated elements of effective helping. The first pertains to the fact that any and all concerns and needs of families must be responded to by the early-intervention practitioner; otherwise, one is likely to communicate a lack of interest and concern regarding the family needs. "To be effective (in work with families), service providers must want to hear what parents have to say and must be truly interested in understanding the family's concerns and needs."[24(p463)] The second pertains to a major role early-intervention practitioners must play in interactions with families. Part H of Public Law 99-457 is explicit in stating that no one person or program should provide all the resources and services a family needs, but that service providers should assist families in accessing needed resources. To assist families, one links them with other support systems that they can mobilize to procure needed resources. Early-intervention practitioners who perform this function help families become more knowledgeable about resources and service options, create opportunities for families to make informed decisions about the assets and limitations of different options, link families with desired resources and services, and promote and enhance the family's acquisition of competencies necessary to mobilize resources to meet needs.

Lastly, both the development and implementation of the IFSP should emphasize promotion of the competence of the family and interdependence with members of the family's community. Competence refers to the capacity to identify needs, assess options for meeting needs, and mobilize resources required to support and strengthen family functioning. Interdependence refers to the joint efforts among family members and between the family and members of their formal and informal social network designed to promote well-being and strengthen the functioning of all network members. If needs are met in a way that promotes acquisition of a family's knowledge and competencies so that there are discernible changes in the family system and their personal social network, the interventions can be considered truly successful.

These four basic but far-reaching principles guide the process of developing and writing IFSPs. A particular format has evolved from the authors' work and guides the development and implementation process.

A format for writing IFSPs

The IFSP form is divided into two parts. Part A includes the following background information:

- the name of the early-intervention practitioner who will function in a number of roles intended to empower families with the knowledge and skills necessary to identify needs and mobilize resources;
- a statement of the child's strengths and current levels of functioning;
- a statement of the family's unique strengths and intrafamily resources; and
- a cumulative record of the specific services, programs, community agencies, and other community support systems and programs that the child and family have employed or are currently using to access resources to meet needs.

Part B of the plan is the working document that guides needs specification and resource mobilization. It includes

- a list of family-identified needs, aspirations, and projects in order of priority;
- a series of statements regarding the sources of support and resources that will be mobilized to meet needs;
- a series of statements regarding the actions that will be taken by the family and early-intervention practitioner to mobilize resources; and
- procedures for evaluating the extent to which needs are met.

The background information section of the IFSP includes data and descriptors useful for depicting unique features of both the child and family and the support systems used to meet child and family needs. Space is provided for recording the child and family's name and the name of the early-intervention practitioner, child behavior and development (strengths and capabilities, current levels of functioning), family functioning style (strengths and capabilities, intrafamily resources), and community support services (informal, formal).

The intervention plan section for the IFSP provides the framework for describing

- what the needs are for the child, siblings, parents, and family;
- who is going to do what to mobilize resources (via intrafamily, informal, community, or formal support);
- what is to be done by the family and the early-intervention practitioner to attain stated intentions; and
- how effective actions are in accomplishing goal attainment and satisfaction.

The intervention plan section of the IFSP is physically formatted in a 28 cm × 43 cm booklet that allows the early-intervention practitioner to keep a running account of the needs, sources of support, and actions taken to mobilize resources to meet needs (Fig 2). The process of writing the plan consists of the following five steps:

1. The date on which the need was identified is recorded. Family-identified needs and projects are recorded continuously as they are identified during interactions with family members. They are recorded on the IFSP in order of priority and reflect the family's desire to take actions necessary to meet needs. Listing needs in this fashion provides a cumulative record of the particular projects and aspirations that constituted the targets of intervention by the family and service provider. The simplicity of this recording system ensures that all concerns are documented, since no elaborate plan needs to be written at this or any point in the IFSP process.

2. A needs statement is written that outlines both what is to occur (process) and what is expected to be accomplished (outcome) as a result of actions to obtain needed resources. Needs, goals, and aspirations are written as "in order to" statements so they are functionally based and easily understood. Something is done in order to have something else achieved or attained (eg, the mother will obtain additional information about her child's genetic disorder in order to learn more about its implications for future development). The present authors have found that both child- and family-level needs can easily be stated in this format. All needs state-

Child____________________ Parent____________________ Early Intervention Practitioner____________________

DATE	NEED STATEMENT	SOURCE OF SUPPORT/RESOURCE	COURSE OF ACTION	EVALUATION DATE					

Fig 2. The physical layout of the intervention plan section of the Individualized Family Support Plan.

ments are phrased in proactive, growth-producing outcomes to reflect the positive stance taken toward children and families. It has been the authors' experience that regardless of the need or specific family situation, all needs can be stated in this manner.

3. The sources of support that will be used to obtain needed resources and the particular aid or assistance that will be procured are specified. The individuals or support systems that will be accessed to obtain the needed resource (aid, assistance, advice), and the particular help or aid that they will provide, are listed as succinctly as possible. To the extent appropriate, the sources of support and resources that are listed include individual family members, personal social network members, and community and formal support systems.

4. Actions that will be taken to mobilize the support sources to obtain needed resources are specified. The steps that will be taken to mobilize resources to meet needs are listed for both the family and early-intervention practitioner. The actions are stated in terms of what will be done by each partner to actualize the plan. Doing so emphasizes shared responsibility (partnership) between the family and early-intervention practitioner. The authors' experience tells them that by stating what each partner will do, the likelihood of resource mobilization occurring in a timely manner is increased considerably.

5. Progress toward resource mobilization in terms of both goal attainment and family satisfaction is evaluated. The method for evaluating the effectiveness of the IFSP assesses the degree to which both actions result in resource mobilization and goal attainment and the family is satisfied with the process and outcome. Each and every contact with the family (eg, face-to-face, phone) is used to evaluate progress toward resource mobilization and goal attainment. The family is simply asked whether or not they have had the opportunity to do a particular step, and how they feel about goal attainment and progress toward the stated intentions. The following rating scale is used for assessing the effectiveness of implementation efforts for each needs statement:

1. Situation changed or worsened; no longer a need, goal, or project.
2. Situation unchanged; still a need, goal, or project.
3. Implementation begun; still a need, goal, or project.
4. Outcome partially attained or accomplished.
5. Outcome accomplished or attained; but not to the family's satisfaction.
6. Outcome mostly accomplished or attained to the family's satisfaction.
7. Outcome completely accomplished or attained to the family's satisfaction.

This simple and relatively straightforward evaluation scheme has proved to have general utility for assessing the effectiveness of the IFSP without the need to develop separate evaluation criteria for each needs statement.

Case example

Table 1 shows an example of both a child-level and family-level needs statement that is written in the format just described. The examples are taken from an actual IFSP written by a program staff member with a mother who had recently become separated from her husband. The mother had 3-year-old and 20-month-old daughters, and was pregnant with her third child. The family became involved in the program because the youngest child had a visual impairment. A total of 16 needs were identified and addressed during a four-month intervention period. The examples shown in Table 1 are representative of the general foci of the collaborative efforts between the family and early-intervention practitioner. The child-level need was identified by the mother because of her concern about not being able to carry her vision-impaired daughter as her pregnancy progressed. Her daughter's ability to pull-to-stand and independently cruise around the room improved within two months after the need was first identified. The family-level need was identified because the family, already living in a crowded apartment, would need additional space once the new infant was born. At the present time, the mother and early-intervention practitioner are continuing to pursue options to meet this need.

BENEFITS AND IMPLICATIONS

The development of the IFSP process described in this article evolved within the context of a number of model-demonstration programs and special projects designed to identify the best ways to support and strengthen family functioning. Both the families and staff who have participated in the development and field testing of the IFSP have reported numerous benefits that are not realized when less flexible and more static approaches are used to develop intervention plans. Several of the comments made by staff who have used the IFSP process and written format have included the following:

- "This approach provides a picture of the partnership relationship between the family and professional."
- "It actually documents what really is important to the family."
- "It keeps me focused on the things that are going on with the family."
- "This approach makes it clear who is in control of making decisions about what is needed by the child and family."

The families who agreed to participate in the field testing of the IFSP approach have reported personal benefits as well. Comments made by these families have included the following:

- "It makes me feel like I'm really accomplishing things for my family."

Table 1. Illustrative examples of Individualized Family Support Plan activities

Child-level activity	*Family-level activity*
1. *Needs identification* 2/1/88 S. will be provided increased opportunities to cruise along furniture to promote independent walking	1. *Needs identification* 2/1/88 Family will explore alternative housing opportunities in order to find larger accommodations for the mother, the children, and new infant
2. *Sources of support and resources* Mother—Physically arrange apartment to encourage cruising Early-intervention practitioner—Provide information regarding intervention strategies Family and friends—Provide encouragement to S. to cruise while providing child care	2. *Sources of support and resources* Family, friends, and neighbors—Information about available apartment or house to rent Newspaper—Classified section on house or apartment rentals Local realty company—Listing of rental housing Public Housing Authority—Information regarding eligibility and availability of public housing
3. *Course of action* *Mother* A. Position furniture so S. can reach without obstacles B. Place toys with sound just beyond her reach to encourage movement to obtain the toys C. Verbally encourage S. to cruise and praise for her attempts D. Demonstrate strategies for family and friends regarding methods to encourage S. to cruise *Early-intervention practitioner* A. Discuss intervention strategies with mother regarding arrangement of furniture and techniques to encourage cruising B. Provide feedback to the mother as she demonstrates techniques C. Demonstrate strategies to other family and friends, as requested by mother	3. *Course of action* *Mother* A. Ask extended family members, friends, and neighbors about their knowledge of available rental housing B. Obtain local newspaper and review listings for available rental housing C. Call local realty company to inquire about listings or available housing for rent *Early-intervention practitioner* A. Will call Public Housing Authority to obtain eligibility information and availability of housing B. Share information with family
4. *Evaluation* 2/15/88 Progress proceeding (3)* 3/1/88 Partially attained (4) 3/15/88 Mostly attained (6) 4/1/88 Accomplished (7)	4. *Evaluation* 3/15/88 Situation unchanged (2) 4/1/88 Progress proceeding (3) 5/10/88 Partially attained (4)

*See text for explanation of ratings.

- "This approach helps focus on the things that my family can do and not what we cannot do."
- "It helps me see who the people are that can help me when I need it."
- "This plan changes as my family's needs change."

Collectively, these comments reflect the fact that the approach to developing and writing IFSPs described in this article yields practical and personal benefits that otherwise might not be realized by other approaches to developing family-level intervention plans. The authors are currently completing an empirical investigation designed to document the increased efficiency of their IFSP process compared to a static framework that had been used prior to the implementation of the more flexible and functional approach to developing and writing family support plans. The results from this study should provide additional support concerning the usefulness of developing IFSPs in the manner described in this article.

• • •

The IFSP approach to identifying and meeting family needs described in this article has been found to be particularly effective in work with families, and represents at least one viable system for developing, implementing, and evaluating family support plans. To be effective in work with families, early-intervention practitioners must be both flexible and functional in the ways in which they identify family concerns and interests and intervene to meet needs. Family support plans must reflect this flexibility and functionality if early-intervention practitioners are to be continually responsive to changes in the family system. Family-level intervention plans that meet these criteria can serve as blueprints for supporting and strengthening family functioning. As both architects and builders, the family and early-intervention practitioner can go about mobilizing support systems to meet needs in ways that enhance parent, family, and child competence. To the extent these outcomes are realized, the intervention efforts may be considered effective.

REFERENCES

1. Hobbs N, Dokecki PR, Hoover-Dempsey KV, et al: *Strengthening Families.* San Francisco, Calif, Jossey-Bass, 1984.
2. Kagan S, Powell D, Weissbourd B, et al (eds): *America's Family Support Programs: Perspectives and Prospects.* New Haven, Conn, Yale University Press, 1987.
3. Pooley LE, Littell JH: *Family Resource Program Builder: Blueprints for Designing and Operating Programs for Parents.* Chicago, Ill, Family Resource Coalition, 1986.
4. Dunst CJ, Trivette CM, Deal AG: *Enabling and Empowering Families: Principles and Guidelines for Practice.* Cambridge, Mass, Brookline Books, 1988.
5. House of Representatives Report 99-860: Education of the Handicapped Act Amendments of 1986, September 1986.

6. Dunst CJ: Helping relationships and enabling and empowering families. Read before the 11th Annual Regional Intervention Program Expansion Conference, Cleveland, Ohio, Oct 23, 1986.
7. Dunst CJ: What is effective helping? Read before the Fifth Biennial National Training Institute of the National Center for Clinical Infant Programs, Washington, DC, Dec 4, 1987.
8. Dunst CJ: Enabling and empowering families: Caveats, considerations and consequences. Read before the Early Intervention: Innovations in Service Delivery Conference, Danbury, Conn, Mar 25, 1988.
9. Dunst CJ, Trivette CM: Enabling and empowering families: Conceptual and intervention issues. *School Psychol Review* 1987;16:443–456.
10. Dunst CJ, Trivette CM: Helping, helplessness, and harm, in Witt J, Elliott S, Gresham F (eds): *Handbook of Behavior Therapy in Education.* New York, Plenum Press, 1988.
11. Rappaport J: In praise of paradox: A social policy of empowerment over prevention. *Am J Community Psychol* 1981;9:1–25.
12. Rappaport J: Terms of empowerment/Exemplars of prevention: Toward a theory for community psychology. *Am J Community Psychol* 1987;15:121–128.
13. Stinnett N, DeFrain J (eds): *Secrets of Strong Families.* New York, Berkley Books, 1985.
14. Dunst CJ: Rethinking early intervention. *Anal Interven Dev Disab* 1985;5:165–201.
15. Dunst CJ, Trivette CM: Social support and positive functioning in families of developmentally, at-risk preschoolers. Read before the symposium "Every Cloud Has a Silver Lining: Successful Adaptations to the Care of a Handicapped Child," held at the Biennial Meeting of the Society for Research in Child Development, Baltimore, Md, Apr 24, 1987.
16. Dunst CJ, Trivette CM: Toward experimental evaluation of the Family, Infant and Preschool Program, in Weiss H, Jacobs F (eds): *Evaluating Family Programs.* New York, Aldine de Gruyter, 1988.
17. Dunst CJ, Leet H, Trivette CM: Family resources, personal well-being, and early intervention. *J Spec Educ* 1988;22:108–116.
18. Bronfenbrenner U: *The Ecology of Human Development: Experiments by Nature and Design.* Cambridge, Mass: Harvard University Press, 1979.
19. Dunst, CJ, Trivette CM: A family systems model of early intervention with handicapped and developmentally at-risk children, in Powell D (ed): *Parent Education and Support Programs: Consequences for Children and Families.* New York, Ablex, to be published.
20. Maple FF: *Shared Decision Making.* Beverly Hills, Calif, Sage, 1977.
21. Shelton TL, Jeppson ES, Johnson BH: *Family-Centered Care for Children with Special Health Care Needs.* Washington, DC, Association for the Care of Children's Health, 1987.
22. McGonigel M, Garland C: The individualized family service plan and the early intervention team: Team and family issues and recommended practices. *Inf Young Children* 1988;1(1):10–21.
23. Dunst CJ, Paget KD: Parent-professional partnerships and family empowerment, in Fine M (ed): *Collaborative Involvement with Parents of Exceptional Children,* to be published.
24. Stoneman Z: Family involvement in early childhood special education programs, in Fallen NH, Umansky W (eds): *Young Children with Special Needs.* Columbus, Ohio, Charles E. Merrill, 1985.

Interactional issues: Infants, parents, professionals

Sally Provence, MD
Senior Research Scientist
Professor Emeritus of Pediatrics and Child Development
Child Study Center
Yale University School of Medicine
New Haven, Connecticut

THE HEIGHTENED emphasis in recent years on the importance of feelings and of relationships with others to the development and well-being of infants and their families is a welcome occurrence. Such renewed attention promises to correct tendencies to overvalue specialized knowledge in one or another area at the expense of a more holistic view, which acknowledges the roles of emotion and of social experience. Infant care professionals cannot understand development or devise the most effective approaches to service without such thinking. Furthermore, because interactions with others, including the concomitant feelings, are part of what professionals are and do, thought must be given to how relationships between infants, parents, and professionals influence the professionals' daily work and its effectiveness.

The steady accumulation of information from research, clinical, and educational practice and the increased participation of users in service planning and delivery have encouraged a reexamination of what makes services beneficial to those who seek or need them. Professionals' perspectives are shifting from narrow to broader views of health and development, and they are more willing to grapple with a more complex approach to assessment and to ways of alleviating developmental delays, handicaps, or behavioral disturbances of infancy and early childhood.

In child development research, too, as Sander[1] has emphasized, there has been a transition from the classical experimental approach, which aims at isolating variables and pursuing linear concepts of causality, toward the study of concurrent and interactive effects of multiple variables, mechanisms of integration, and the formulation of nonlinear concepts of causality. Sander argues persuasively that such research is badly needed to enrich the empirical base from which professionals can construct a more astute conceptualization of the developmental process. These conceptual advances will aid practitioners in their commitment to early intervention that helps prevent or alleviate developmental deviations when either the infant or the caregiving environment is dysfunctional.

The basic understanding of children and guidelines for practice that each practitioner brings to his or her daily work come from state-of-the-art knowledge of development and behavior drawn from a variety of studies. Healthy children have been studied in favorable environments and in noxious environments, and children who suffer from inborn or acquired mental or physical handicaps have been studied in nurturing, supportive environments and in unfavorable environments. Other studies focus on individual differences, and still others delineate common

Inf Young Children 1990; 3(1): 1–7

patterns of development and behavior, including behavioral and test norms. It is known that handicaps can be single or multiple; that risk factors may be transitory or cumulative; that multiple risk factors are associated with less good outcomes than single risk factors[2]; and that biologically vulnerable infants are likely to suffer more in environments that do not meet their needs reasonably well than are robust, healthy infants.[3] Two concepts—that infants influence the behavior of their caregivers[4] and that they have some ability to cope with stress[5]—have modified the view of infants as totally helpless and have turned attention to how inherent or acquired adaptive capacities can be enhanced.

This article paints in broad strokes a view of interaction, most centrally parent–child interaction, and some aspects of its significance for practice. In addition to the focus on parent and child, two other aspects of interaction are considered: interaction as a factor in the developmental process and interaction of professionals with parents and child as a determinant of effectiveness of service.

INTERACTION AND DEVELOPMENT

Development of the individual child is a process characterized by the interaction of biological and environmental factors. Lines or domains of development, whether focused on language, motility, cognition, affect (or emotion), social relatedness, or levels of organization of experience, are viewed as interdependent. The concept that influences are multiple, complex, and interacting, while mind boggling in scope and a challenge to any person's imperfect capacity to study or even to keep in mind, is of singular importance for continued progress toward greater understanding and through that to greater effectiveness in developing and delivering services.

THE CHILD

Early childhood specialists of many philosophical and theoretical persuasions share the view that the child's human relationships are crucially important for his or her physical, mental, and emotional development and for his or her full participation in society and culture. Whether stated in the language of psychoanalytic object relations theory, attachment theory, Erikson's psychosocial theory, social learning theory, or one of several philosophies of early childhood education, what goes on between the child and those closest to him or her is acknowledged as critical in its influence on current and future development.

The infant is biologically predisposed to, ready for, and attracted to social interaction with caregivers from birth. Under average conditions, this readiness is coordinated with the responsiveness of adults to the infant's needs and with tendencies of their own to protect and nurture. The unfolding of the genetically social character of the human individual within the social environment at each phase of development has been traced, for example, in Erikson's[6] psychosocial theory.

Erikson's concept of mutuality specifies that there is a crucial coordination between the individual and his or her social environment and that this coordination is mutual. Studies[4] of the origins of reciprocity in maternal–infant interaction illustrate the mutuality of the adaptation between parent and infant. Societal and cultural influences on infant development are transmitted and mediated by the caretakers.

Much of what experts currently agree on regarding the significance of infant–adult interaction for the child's development has been summarized by Provence and Naylor[7] as follows: The benevolence, reliability, and continuity of the nurturing persons are important because such care stimulates specific dimensions of development. Interaction with caregivers influences in important ways such mental functions as the child's ability to discriminate between things and persons in the environment; to distinguish between the outside world and the inner world of sensation, thought, and feeling; and to take interest in objects and activities. Motility, perception, speech, intelligence, and the ability to organize experience are enhanced or impeded according to the nature of the psychosocial environment. The child's perception and intelligence are involved in his or her relationships with others from the beginning. For example, the infant's ability first to recognize the mother and to read nonverbal cues and later to understand speech involves significant cognitive elements, while emotional tone and motivation are drawn from the highly personalized interaction between them.

Relationships with others also profoundly influence the development of coping strategies and adaptive behavior and the formation of stable psychological defenses. Experiences of mastery, which influence motivation, identity, and self-esteem, flourish in environments where children are stimulated and given the opportunity to use emerging skills in a protective and distinctly affectionate environment. The child's development and expression of affects illustrates the mutual influences of inborn and experiential factors. Research regarding the emotions has been reemphasized and extended in recent years.[8–12] As Emde and colleagues[11] note, affects are recognized as continuous aspects of people's lives, as vital ingredients for social relatedness, and as inseparably linked with social experience. Moreover, from an adaptational point of view, affects have a social signalling function from the beginning of life that serves survival. This is in part what Erikson has put so felicitously:

> The weakness of the newborn . . . is truly relative. While far removed from any measure of mastery over the physical world, newborn man is endowed with an appearance and with responses which appeal to the tending adults' tenderness and make them wish to attend to his needs; which arouse concern in those who are concerned with his well being; and which, in making adults care, stimulate their caretaking. . . .[13(pp114–115)]

Varied forms of expression of comfort, discomfort, pleasure, and protest are recognizable from early infancy by parents and other caregivers, as well as by investigators. While the range and variety of emotions and their expression increase in complexity over time, the occurrence of facial expressions recognized universally as expressing basic emotions operates from birth onward. They are rooted in biology but also are subject to social learning, beginning with the earliest reciprocal interchanges and transactions with caregivers.

In one sense infant affects are shaped by the social environment, and in another the preadapted structures infants bring with them influence the environment, most importantly their caregivers, in significant ways. Greenspan and Greenspan[14] have spoken of the relationship between parents and child as "the essential partnership," a characterization that captures the vital importance for both parent and child of the complex exchanges that take place between them as they meet the emotional challenges of infancy and childhood.

Affective interchanges nourish the developing relationship for infant and for parent. Even when they are not perceived as the center of an interaction or of an identified skill or function, they are its accompaniment, as vital and ever present as the air we breathe.

THE PARENTS

Any consideration of interactional issues requires as much understanding as possible about attitudes and behavior of parents and the complex dynamic social system of the family. Dealing with the richness and complexity of the family system is beyond the scope of this article. But from the perspective of parent–child interaction and of parenthood as a developmental process, a number of points have particular relevance.

Pregnancy and prospective parenthood have been called a normal developmental crisis[15,16] that imposes new adaptive tasks. As a major turning point in life, these events bring about changes in personality equilibrium even in relatively healthy persons; unresolved conflicts may emerge from the past, or mastery of adult developmental task and phases may improve.

The attitudes and behavior of parents toward parenthood and toward the infant are influenced by many factors in their previous lives, including their own family and cultural experience; current realities in their life situation, including socioeconomic and interpersonal factors; and the characteristics of the child.

The process of adaptation to parenthood is powerfully stimulated by contact with the newborn, and parental attitudes are continuously influenced by the child's growth and development. The child's changing needs and behavior stimulate changing attitudes and behavior in parents. A mother who delights in her infant may react with irritation or anxiety when he or she moves toward greater autonomy and independence. The opposite may also occur: A child who has become more independent or begun to talk may give great pleasure to a parent who did not enjoy the younger, more dependent infant. Other well-known sensitive issues for parents related to their child's development are negativism, separation, sphincter control, aggressive behavior, and sexual curiosity. These account for acute parent–child conflict at times. But they also provide opportunities for parents to resolve their own feelings and internal conflicts about these sensitive areas and to reach a new level of integration and harmony.

Parental attitudes and thus behavior toward the child are determined largely by the parent's personality and the meaning of the child to him or her. It is a favorable sign when parents can adapt reasonably well not only to the reality of the child they have, but also to the changing characteristics and needs that are inherent in development. For most parents, the satisfactions, pleasures, and fulfillment associated with nurturing the young outweigh the discomforts of worry, loss of sleep, and other stresses. Even when things are difficult in the short term, most parents experience more good times than bad, more joy than pain, and more satisfaction than frustration. The bonds of love established between adult and child make many things possible and cause strengths to emerge or be built that parents did not know they had. These important processes of growth occur and are fed by the hundreds and thousands of interactions between parents and child as they live their lives together in an intensely personal, emotionally rich, and intimate way.

When one views parenthood as a challenging and potentially difficult stage of life but as one offering a new identity and sense of fulfillment, enhanced self-esteem, and pleasure, the situation of the parents of an infant with a chronic illness or handicap is especially poignant. Expectations for a healthy, well-functioning, robust child must be modified. The brightness of parental hopes and dreams is dimmed by an often cruel reality. In such situations, parents of a vulnerable child become vulnerable, too. The weaknesses or vulnerabilities of the infant may be magnified by parental responses. Conversely, the infant's vulnerabilities or handicaps may activate resources in the parents that enable them to respond with sensitive attention to special needs, thus optimizing the child's potential. Developmental accomplishments that are small when compared with healthy children become major victories and sources of pride and pleasure. The process in parents of coming to terms with their sadness, disappointment, and often anger is a challenge requiring all of their capacities for recovery and adaptation.

The same process of adaptation is experienced by parents whose disappointment is not because of a vulnerability or an identified deficit in their infant, but because it is a girl when a boy is wanted, or arrives at the wrong time, or is too active or too inactive, or reminds them too much of a figure from the past, or is of a temperament that does not fit well with the personalities and abilities of the parents. Granted the singular importance of parent–child relationships, how do professionals learn to understand, to offer support, and to respond to the need for assistance when problems ensue? As investigators and as practitioners, infant care professionals rely on multiple sources of data. They seek information from parents about their child and about themselves. They observe parent and child interacting in a variety of settings, either naturalistic or fashioned for a specific purpose. They look closely at the child's developmental level and behavior through formal and informal methods of assessment. They ask for information from others who know the child well.

In some instances, it does not require an expert eye to observe signs of troubled relationships (eg, the inactivity and psychological unavailability of a depressed mother and her apathetic or irritable infant). Indicators of difficulty in reciprocal communication and mutual adaptation are often more subtle, yet observable when looking closely. Reasonable inferences about the inner life of the infant and the parent–child relationship from surface behavior are often possible but are sometimes impossible.

Despite the fact that professionals can learn a great deal about an infant's development by careful observation of behavior, not everything of vital importance that goes on in development and between two persons is expressed in observable behavior. An awareness of this fact is a safeguard against practitioners' deluding themselves by oversimplifying complex issues. Still, careful observation of parent–child interaction, especially in the preverbal years, provides information that can lead to the refinement of assessment procedures and the creation of reasonable individualized responses to the need for assistance.[17,18] Thus, observation of parent–child interaction is a skill to be sought by infant and early childhood specialists.

THE PROFESSIONALS

As practitioners serving infants and parents, whether as clinicians, educators, or providers of substitute child care, professionals do their work in a social context. Achieving excellence begins, of course, with commitment to the mastery of the content and methods of the various disciplines. The use of the human, socially anchored aspect of self in daily work is part of that excellence—that is, the joining of the science with what has been called the art of practice. Some attributes of the excellent practitioner are not recognized as part of the science. But empathy, warmth, courtesy, and attentive interest toward child and parent enhance the trust in the practitioner and facilitate diagnosis and the formation of a therapeutic alliance on behalf of the child. In the absence of feelings of confidence and trust, without mutual respect, and without the development, however gradual, of a working partnership between parents and practitioner, it is unlikely that the goal of providing comprehensive services of high quality for children will be realized.

If one accepts the idea that effective interviewing is a necessary component of medical, developmental, and psychosocial diagnosis, then the nature of the interaction among those involved assumes great importance. Practitioners must create an atmosphere in which parents feel supported in a difficult experience and respected for their knowledge and concern. Empathy, warmth, courtesy, and respectful attention as well as skillful questioning and sensitive listening—all essentially interactional—are major determinants of the efficacy of diagnosis, treatment, and individualized service plans.

Green,[19] who pleads for an expansion of the traditional focus on the medical complaint, advises pediatric professionals that patients want their physicians to care about them. Continuity of care in health services is generally known to improve quality and efficient use. Continuity and caring, as well as competence in providing health, social, and educational services, have been found to characterize the programs that have made a substantial difference in outcome for disadvantaged families.[7,20–23]

Interviewing skills, including the awareness that the practitioner's attitudes and feelings influence assessment and treatment, have received insufficient attention in many child-focused disciplines. The need for skillful interviewing in work with children as well as parents requires an expansion of traditional training for infancy and early childhood professionals.

Some principles of effective interviewing and an illustration are found in recently published guidelines for screening and assessment.[23] General goals for the interviewer include the following:

- to create a comfortable and benevolent atmosphere in which parents feel supported and enabled to participate actively in the process;
- to develop, not through a mechanistic question-and-answer process but through sensitive questioning, listening, and observing, a picture of parental concerns, the natural history of the problems they describe, and the events and feelings surrounding them;
- to assess the family as a child-rearing environment for the child in question;
- to obtain a full picture of the health and development of the child;
- to engage regularly during the evaluation process in exchange of significant information with other staff members who see the child and family; and
- to share with parents what is learned about the child and recommendations for further evaluation or intervention.

The guidelines list 24 conventionally used subject areas for evaluating a young child that include such diverse factors as health, environment, pregnancy, labor and delivery, feeding, sleep, activity and motor development, language, play, feelings, social experiences, fears, and other developmental and behavioral domains.[23]

The guidelines advise professionals to help parents prepare their child for the evaluation process. The professional must be flexible enough to elicit enough information to guide the assessment while being able to follow the leads that emerge during the interview. It is very important to recognize that relevant information from the parents will continue to emerge as the assessment proceeds and the working relationship is forged. From the very first contact parents and child have with the individual practitioner, team, or agency and throughout the entire process, the interactions among all concerned will either facilitate or impede the provision and efficient use of high-quality services.

• • •

Individual practitioners and teams, then, must give high priority to refining skills that enable valid assessment and effective treatment or preventive intervention programs. With so much to learn from so many sources, professionals must devote much effort to integrating knowledge and practice.

REFERENCES

1. Sander L. Investigation of the infant and its caregiving environment as a biological system. In: Greenspan SI, Pollock GH, eds. *The Course of Life: Psychoanalytic Contributions Toward Understanding Personality Development.* Washington, DC: National Institute of Mental Health; 1980:1.
2. Greenspan SI. Theoretical perspectives on research regarding psychopathology and preventive intervention in infancy. In Greenspan SI, Weider S, Nover R, Lieberman A, Lourie R, Robinson M, eds. *Infants in Multirisk Families: Case Studies in Preventive Intervention Clinical Infant Reports.* Madison, Conn: International Universities Press; 1987; (No. 3).
3. Sameroff AJ, Seifer R, Zax M. Early development of children at risk for emotional disorder: Monograph of the Society for Research in Child Development. 1982;47(No. 7).
4. Brazelton TB, Koslowski B, Main M. The origins of reciprocity. In: Lewis M, Rosenblum LA, eds. *The Effect of the Infant on Its Caregivers.* New York, NY: Wiley; 1974.
5. Murphy, LB. Coping, vulnerability and resilience in childhood. In: Coelho GV, Hamburg DA, Adams JE, eds. *Coping and Adaptation.* New York, NY: Basic Books; 1974.
6. Erikson EH. Identity and the life cycle: Psychological issues monograph. 1959;1(No. 1).
7. Provence S, Naylor A. *Working with Disadvantaged Parents and Their Children: Scientific and Practice Issues.* New Haven, Conn: Yale University Press; 1983.
8. Izard CE. Emotions as motivators: An evolutionary-developmental perspective. In: Dienstbier R, ed. *Nebraska Symposium on Motivation.* Lincoln, Neb: University of Nebraska Press; 1979.
9. Lewis M, Michalson L. *Childrens' Emotions and Moods.* New York, NY: Plenum Press; 1983.
10. Emde R. Toward a psychoanalytic theory of affect. In: Greenspan SI, Pollock GH, eds. *The Course of Life: Psychoanalytic Contributions Toward Understanding Personality Development.* Washington, DC: Government Printing Office; 1980;1.
11. Emde R, Gaensbauer T, Harmon R. Emotional expression in infancy: A biobehavioral study: Psychological issues monograph. 1976;10.
12. Tronick E. *Affect, Cognition and Communication.* Baltimore, Md: University Park Press; 1982.
13. Erikson EH. Human strength and the cycle of generations. In: *Insight and Responsibility.* New York, NY: Norton; 1964.
14. Greenspan SI, Greenspan NT. *The Essential Partnership.* New York, NY: Viking; 1989.
15. Bibring GL. Some considerations of the psychological procures in pregnancy. In: *The Psychoanalytic Study of the Child.* New York, NY: International Universities Press; 1959;14.

16. Naylor AK. Some determinants of parent–infant relationships. In: Dittman L, ed. *What We Can Learn from Infants.* Washington, DC: National Association for the Education of Young Children; 1970.

17. Bromwich R. *Working With Parents and Infants: An Interactional Approach.* Baltimore, Md: University Park Press; 1981.

18. Barnard KE, LeBaron K. McCarthy AM, et al. *Blueprint for Assessment Diagnosis and Treatment in Parent-Child Nursing.* Seattle, Wash: University of Washington, NCAST Publication; 1986.

19. Green M. The pediatric interview and history. In: *Pediatric Diagnosis.* 3rd ed. Philadelphia, Pa: W.B. Saunders; 1980.

20. Schorr LB. The lessons of successful programs. In: *Within Our Reach: Breaking The Cycle of Disadvantages.* New York, NY: Anchor Press; 1988.

21. Olds DL, Henderson CR, Tatelbaum R, Chamberlin R. Improving the delivery of prenatal care and outcomes of pregnancy: A randomized trial of nurse home visitation. *Pediatrics.* 1986;77:16–28.

22. Seitz V, Rosenbaum LK, Apfel NH. Effects of family support intervention: A ten-year follow-up. *Child Dev.* 1985;53:376–391.

23. Meisels SJ, Provence S. *Screening and Assessment: Guidelines for Identifying Young Disabled and Developmentally Vulnerable Children and Their Families.* Washington, DC: National Center for Clinical Infant Programs; 1989.

Early intervention with culturally diverse families of infants and toddlers with disabilities

Sam Chan, PhD
Multicultural Training Director
University Affiliated Program
Center for Child Development and
Developmental Disorders
Childrens Hospital Los Angeles
Los Angeles, California

AS THE UNITED STATES enters the final decade of this century, it is undergoing one of the most significant demographic shifts in its history, By the year 2000, one third of the projected US population will consist of African-Americans, American Indians, Asian Pacifics, Latinos, and other people of color.[1] Moreover, as the white American population continues to grow older, it will also achieve minority status in numerous regions throughout the country. For example, shortly after the turn of this century, the white population in the state of California will be in the minority. In fact, the school-age population of California has already passed this benchmark; members of ethnic minorities now constitute a majority of the state's public school students.[2]

This accelerated growth is largely attributable to the continuing influx of millions of immigrants and refugees as well as to the relatively high birth rates among those populations. The newly arrived populations are characterized by predominantly Asian and Latino families who speak little or no English and have young children, including significant numbers of children with developmental special needs. They, in turn, are joined by dramatically increasing numbers of African-American and other native-born minority children who are at risk or disabled because of perinatal substance abuse, prenatal infection, poor maternal nutrition, prematurity, low birth weight, and other adverse conditions associated with rising poverty and destructive social forces (*News Digest.* 1987;9:2).

In the midst of these population trends and crises are programs and service delivery systems attempting to implement the policy mandates of Public Law 99-457. As one of the required components of Part H, Early Intervention Program for Handicapped Infants and Toddlers, the individualized family service plan (IFSP) "represents the cornerstone of the entire system of early intervention services."[3(pvii)] Among the principles underlying the IFSP process are the following: 1) "Early intervention systems and strategies must reflect a respect for the racial, ethnic, and cultural diversity of families, [and] 2) early intervention serv-

The programs described in this article were supported by grants from the California State Department of Developmental Services and the U.S. Department of Education, Office of Special Education and Rehabilitative Services. The author acknowledges the staff and families who participated in these programs and the following collaborating agencies: Asian Community Mental Health Services, Chinatown Child Development Center, Union of Pan Asian Communities, El Arca Human Services Corporation, and Protection and Advocacy, Inc.

Inf Young Children 1990; 3(2): 78–87

ices should be flexible, accessible, and responsive to family needs."[3(p6)] Unfortunately, these principles do not translate easily into comprehensive, family-centered, community-based early intervention for *all* infants and toddlers with disabilities.

The effectiveness of early intervention programs that serve multicultural populations "rests heavily upon the sensitivity, understanding, and respect paid to the specific cultural, familial, and individual diversity involved."[4(p18)] However, acknowledgment, awareness, and good intentions will not in themselves produce culturally and linguistically appropriate services for selected populations. The previously described population trends and characteristics have clearly exacerbated the persistent problem of multiple barriers that inhibit access to needed services and information. These barriers include a lack of language-appropriate informational materials concerning resources, rights, and responsibilities for non–English-speaking individuals. This lack is compounded by an acute shortage of trained bilingual, bicultural personnel among provider agencies and the lack of culturally responsive service models that systematically address relevant cultural orientations and behaviors that affect service utilization. Furthermore, outreach methods employed by agencies serving culturally diverse infants and young children with disabilities and their families are often inadequate.

Among these barriers, the lack of qualified bilingual, bicultural personnel is part of a more general shortage of personnel for the provision of early intervention services that has reached crisis proportions.[5] Such shortages have reinforced the significance of another essential component of Public Law 99-457 policy mandates—the establishment of a comprehensive system of personnel development. This component coupled with the IFSP requirement supports the provision of training and information to families of children with disabilities to promote their meaningful involvement in the process of planning, implementing, and evaluating needed services. Corresponding federally funded parent training and information projects have placed emphasis on serving members of groups who have traditionally been underrepresented.[6] Education and training programs for culturally diverse parents are thus viewed as essential means of promoting family access to needed services and of increasing parental involvement and advocacy in the formulation of policies and development of programs for infants and young children with disabilities.

HISTORICAL OVERVIEW

For the past 6 years, the University-Affiliated Program (UAP) at Childrens' Hospital Los Angeles has collaborated with a number of community-based agencies and organizations to establish statewide projects serving selected Asian, African-American, and Latino populations. Supported through state and federal grants, the Asian and Hispanic Parent Education/Training Project and the Mutlicultural Training-of-Trainers Project addressed the critical need for culturally and linguistically appropriate parent-training models and materials. The projects were designed to enable parents to participate more effectively with professionals in meeting the needs of their children with disabilities and to further empower them to assume leadership roles in their respective ethnic communities.

ASIAN AND HISPANIC PARENT EDUCATION/TRAINING PROJECT

As the first statewide program of its kind, the Asian and Hispanic Parent Education/Training Project was designed to develop and implement a model of comprehensive parent education for Asian and Latino immigrants who speak little or no English and who have developmentally disabled children.

Population

A total of 80 adult family members representing 57 children with developmental disabilities participated in the program. The respective Northern and Southern California program sites served Chinese-speaking families (in the San Francisco and East Bay areas) and Korean- and Spanish-speaking families (in Los Angeles). The majority of families were recent immigrants (less than 5 years in the United States) and the parents' educational levels varied from no formal education to college or university degrees (more than 75% of parents were at least high school graduates). The children ranged in age from 3 months to 12 years (mean age, 5 years). They had primary diagnoses of cerebral palsy, mental retardation, epilepsy, autism, neurologic disorders, and/or related conditions. Most of the children were mentally retarded, including 15 with Down syndrome.

Staff

The principal project staff recruited to serve the respective ethnic parent groups consisted of bilingual and bicultural training coordinators and parent facilitators. These staff members were originally selected on the basis of their potential for establishing successful rapport and working relationships with parent-participants and for serving as effective group facilitators. They had experience working with parent organizations and possessed strong leadership skills. They also demonstrated a high level of sensitivity and versatility in responding effectively to the diverse nationalities, dialects, cultural orientations, educational levels, and social class backgrounds of the parents who ultimately participated in the program. Parent facilitators were recent immigrants and parents of developmentally disabled children; thus, they were particularly aware of the unique life experiences and traditional coping styles of various immigrant families with children with disabilities.

The training coordinators, assisted by parent facilitators, were responsible for implementing each of the major project objectives:

- outreach and recruitment (publicizing the parent education program and identifying parent-participants),
- conducting systematic parent needs assessments,
- developing the parent education program curricula and materials,
- collecting and evaluating outcome data, and
- providing follow-up support and training to parent-participants.

Together they served as team trainers and coleaders in conducting their parent groups.

The training coordinators and parent facilitators received preliminary training relevant to implementation of the parent education curricula. This training addressed the following subjects:

- adult learning principles,
- effective teaching modalities,
- communication and leadership skills,
- group process variables,
- culture-specific group interaction and participation factors,
- curriculum format considerations, and
- guidelines for invited speakers on various topics who would appear throughout the first series.

Model description

Outreach and needs assessment

A variety of parent-participant recruitment strategies were used among the respective project sites. Corresponding outreach activities consisted primarily of soliciting referrals from service provider representatives of various community agencies and from allied health professionals serving the targeted client populations. At selected sites, more extensive outreach efforts entailed dissemination of project information through articles and announcements in various agency newsletters, ethnic newspapers, and television programs and through presentations to community organizations.

Upon indicating an initial interest in participating in the program, individual parents were personally contacted by staff who arranged and conducted home visits. During home visits, a questionnaire was informally administered to the parents to obtain information about family background, the child's disabling condition (history and current parental perceptions), services and/or support received and needed, and parental expectations for the child. Parents were also asked to complete a needs assessment survey in which they rated potential parent curriculum topics in terms of their degree of interest and their specific information needs.

The parents' needs assessments yielded valuable information that was subsequently incorporated into the development of curriculum topics for each respective site. The majority of parents desired objective information about their child's specific disabling condition, particularly with respect to etiology, associated characteristics, and corresponding needs. Parents at each site were also interested in acquiring skills to promote their child's development in various domains, as well as information about rights, resources, and effective utilization of available services. Coping emotionally with a child with a developmental disability and reducing family stress were also identified as important topics, and the presentation of these concerns during the training series had a profound impact on facilitating increased group identification, cohesiveness, and participation.

Curriculum development

Data obtained from the needs assessments served to assist the staff in prioritizing topic areas and were incorporated into the curriculum development process. Pertinent written materials and handouts were designed to be straightforward and practical in content and were prepared in Chinese, Korean, and Spanish, Existing English-language materials were adapted for various topics and modified to be compatible with the unique cultural, linguistic, and learning characteristics of each group of parents. Simple literal translation of these materials was avoided.

Various educational and training formats were also developed. Efforts were made to minimize didactic, lecture-oriented presentations; thus, respective presenters for each session were given guidelines for conducting relatively brief presentations. They were also given sample curriculum materials and information about the characteristics and relevant needs and concerns of the children and parents they were to address. The primary focus of each session was on experiential learning through participant discussion, personal reflection, disclosure, question–answer exchanges, and group problem solving. Corresponding teaching and group facilitation techniques were thus used to sustain participant interest and active involvement in each session.

Implementation

The parent education curricula were implemented at each site throughout an initial 10- to 11-session series of consecutive weekly meetings (each 2-3 hours in duration). Session topics included

- the medical and genetic aspects of developmental disabilities,
- an overview of child development principles,
- improvement of the child's motor, cognitive, language, social, and self-help skills,
- behavior management,
- stress and coping with a disabled child,
- legal rights and responsibilities,

- community resources, and
- advocacy strategies.

The sessions were conducted in the parents' respective native languages. Most of the invited presenters and parent consultants were bilingual and thus able to conduct their presentations and discussions in Chinese (Cantonese/Mandarin dialects), Korean, or Spanish; the project staff served as skilled translators for the English-speaking presenters. Corresponding written materials in the various languages were also distributed to the parent-participants.

New parent-participants were recruited for a second 10- to 11-session series conducted at each site. In addition, bilingual and bicultural service providers representing various disciplines and agencies were invited to join selected groups. They assumed roles as participant observers and trainees so as to experience directly the implementation of the project model and to acquire further skills in developing and conducting similar parent groups.

Program outcomes

Throughout both parent education series, weekly telephone or personal contact with individual parent-participants by the training coordinators and parent facilitators served to enhance parental involvement in each successive session. Consistently good participant attendance (ranging from 80%–100%) was maintained at each site. The training coordinators also engaged in an ongoing evaluation process with the parent facilitators whereby their respective group facilitation skills were assessed for each session. The parent facilitators acquired increasingly sophisticated skills with respect to stimulating participant discussion, sustaining parent interest, motivating follow-through on various recommendations, and creating an atmosphere that engendered mutual trust, openness, and support.

The impact of the program on the parent-participants was highly significant at a number of different levels. One of the most noteworthy developments in each of the sites was the accelerated growth in group cohesiveness, collective problem solving, personalized sharing of experiences and conflicts, and emotional support. Parents who were originally observed to be relatively isolated, nonverbal, reserved, or experiencing significant personal difficulties soon participated actively in the group and, in selected cases, were reported by outside agency staff to also be more actively and positively involved in their children's case management.

Specific individual behavioral changes were further reported by the parents themselves and observed by staff and associated service providers. Parents indicated, for example, that the program had prompted them to engage in more frequent and systematic stimulation of their children with respect to motor, cognitive, language, and social development, and that they observed corresponding improvements in their children's functioning. A number of parents also reported positive changes in the areas of teaching self-help skills and managing problem behaviors.

Some parents further stated that the program helped them to gain valuable insights into the specific nature and possible causes of their children's disabilities and corresponding needs. This in turn enabled them to develop realistic expectations and to educate and support other family members (particularly spouses and older siblings) in gaining similar perspectives. By encouraging parents to develop more positive attitudes and by fostering more effective family dynamics, the program was influential in facilitating the participants' acquisition of improved personal coping, parenting, and advocacy skills. Consequently, many succeeded in overcoming feelings of being stigmatized and ashamed, as well as overcoming the isolation that they had previously experienced.

Follow-up support and program development

A number of parents received individual follow-up assistance from the project staff with respect to obtaining various support services for their children. Many parents were more aware of their children's specific needs, appropriate community resources, their rights, and methods of accessing various service delivery systems as a direct result of their participation in the program. They thus served as effective advocates for themselves and their children and as highly motivated "partners" of the project staff in seeking supportive services in an increasingly self-reliant manner. This partnership further evolved in collaborative endeavors to develop ongoing support networks among project alumni. At each site, many of the original parent-participants joined the second-series parent groups for selected sessions, to share their expertise and experiences and to provide support to the new participants. Moreover, parents succeeded in maintaining personal relationships with one another as well as informal group affiliations that led to more systematic efforts to secure the additional resources needed to continue their educational and support activities.

The development of curriculum materials in the participants' respective languages and the documentation of corresponding training methodologies also represented a unique contribution to the field, as such materials were previously unavailable in many subject areas. This lack of adequate resources has limited the ability of developmental service providers to address the information and service needs of various non–English-speaking Asian and Latino families. The broad-based dissemination of project materials thus served to augment existing limited resources while prompting parents, advocates, and providers to develop similar programs in their respective communities.

One other major accomplishment of the project was the strengthening of interagency and organizational networks throughout the state in an effort to address systematically the needs of undeserved populations. The corresponding collaboration among various community leaders and agency and organization representatives resulted in statewide planning efforts that continued to evolve in a coordinated and sequential manner. The ultimate product of such efforts was the successful establishment of a federally funded project of national significance, the Multicultural Training-of-Trainers Project.

MULTICULTURAL TRAINING-OF-TRAINERS PROJECT

The primary goal of the Multicultural Training-of-Trainers (MTOT) Project was to provide training and information to ethnic minority parents to enable them to participate more effectively with professionals in meeting the educational needs of their children with disabilities. The MTOT Project was specifically directed toward the establishment of culturally and linguistically appropriate training-of-trainers programs. These programs were designed to provide teams of parents and service providers with group organization and leadership training. MTOT Project parent-provider teams subsequently served to organize, develop, and conduct parent training programs in their respective communities. The project further served to disseminate corresponding training-of-trainers models and to facilitate the development of local and statewide parent and professional organizations, networks, and coalitions.

Population

A total of over 400 parents participated in the community-based parent training programs that were conducted by parent-provider teams. Targeted ethnic groups and geographic locations included the same populations previously served through the Asian and Hispanic Parent Education/Training Project, as well as Chinese and African-American parents (in Los Angeles) and Vietnamese parents (in Los Angeles and San Diego). Nearly all the Asian and Latino parents were foreign born and spoke little or no English. Whereas the majority of parents had received 6 to 12 years of formal education (30% were college graduates), a significant number (25%) had either less than 6 years or no formal education. The over 300 children and youths within the families served by the project ranged in age from less than 1 year to 21 years (mean age, 10 years). They were characterized by a full range of disabilities that warranted early intervention and special education and related services. The largest subgroups of children were those who were mentally retarded (27%) or who had orthopedic or physical disabilities (22%).

Staff

Bilingual and bicultural training coordinators were hired for the various MTOT Project sites. The training coordinators were foreign born and fully proficient in the native languages (Chinese, Korean, Vietnamese, Spanish) of their respective countries of origin. Most had also acquired practical experience in implementing relevant parent-training models. Among their responsibilities, the recruitment, training, and supervision of parent trainers were most critical.

The parent trainers recruited at each site were selected on the basis of their ethnic community affiliations, native language proficiency, experience as a parent of a child with a disability, ability to serve as an effective group leader and parent advocate, and motivation and commitment to assume such a role. Many of the 40 parent trainers who were recruited had previously participated in the series of workshops conducted through the Asian and Hispanic Parent Education/Training Project. Some of these project alumni had also received training and served as parent facilitators for their respective parent groups. The parent trainers were primarily responsible for recruiting parent-participants for their respective community-based training programs and then organizing and facilitating monthly parent-training workshops.

Service providers representing diverse disciplines and a variety of agencies serving children with disabilities and their families were recruited to serve as members of the parent-provider teams. Most of the providers were bilingual and bicultural and had previously acquired varying levels of parent-training experience. Their principal responsibility within the MTOT Project was to provide administrative consultation and technical assistance to the parent trainer as he or she developed monthly community-based parent training workshops.

Parent trainer-service provider teams for each site received initial group training consisting of three 6-hour workshops. The specific content of the team training varied according to previously identified information and skill needs of parent trainers and service providers. However, the principal subject areas addressed were similar, including

- information about specific disabilities,
- family coping issues,
- normalization principles,
- legal rights and responsibilities,
- community resources,
- advocacy skills and strategies,
- effective parent-professional communication and collaboration (including relevant cultural considerations), and
- group organization, process, and facilitation.

The training sessions were generally conducted in the native languages of the parent trainers. A variety of training formats was utilized, including individual and panel presentations, media, role-playing, experiential learning exercises, brainstorming, small group discussions, and interactive parent–professional mutual awareness and problem-solving activities.

Model description

Upon completion of the initial team training, parent trainers and service providers engaged in intensive efforts to organize their respective community-based parent-training programs. Each of 30 parent trainer/service provider teams was responsible for recruiting approximately 10 parents of children with disabilities (from birth to 21 years old). The information and training needs of these parents were assessed individually, and corresponding 2- to 3-hour monthly workshops were subsequently conducted for each community-based group throughout a 6-month period. The organization and composition of specific groups at each site ultimately varied according to different participant membership criteria, such as the agency affiliation of the parents, the geographic location, or the specific disability or age range of the children.

Outreach and needs assessment

A variety of parent-participant recruitment strategies were employed at each site. Some teams recruited parents directly from within the respective agencies with which they were affiliated, including regional centers for the developmentally disabled and community-based early childhood (infant/toddler) intervention programs, serving predominantly African-American, Chinese, or Latino families. Broader-based community outreach methods (such as those described in the previous section of this article) were employed in the recruitment of participants at other sites.

Previously developed parent questionnaires and needs assessment surveys were completed for each participating family. The potential workshop topic preferences for parents of younger children, in particular, were very similar to those identified by parents who had participated in the Asian and Hispanic Parent Education/Training Project.

Curriculum development

The selection and development of appropriate curriculum materials for each parent group was an ongoing process in which the parent trainers participated directly. Pertinent written materials and handouts had previously been developed and translated into Chinese, Korean, and Spanish as part of the Asian and Hispanic Parent Education/Training Project. These and additional materials were also translated into Vietnamese.

Implementation

A total of 180 community-based workshops were conducted at the various sites. The workshop topics for each group reflected the previously determined participant preferences. Among the most popular topics were

- the nature and causes of specific disabilities,
- promotion of cognitive and language development,
- family stress and coping,
- participation in the individualized planning process, and
- service rights and benefits.

The workshops were conducted in the parents' respective native languages.

Program outcomes

The parent-participants described a number of principal benefits they received. Among them was the profoundly positive impact of meeting and interacting regularly with parents (including many fathers) who spoke the same language, had similar cultural backgrounds, and experienced similar needs, problems, and concerns. Opportunities to express related feelings and receive mutual support served to reduce emotional stress and the earlier sense of guilt, shame, depression, and isolation which was frequently disclosed by many parents. Another major benefit was the opportunity to receive information and written materials in their native languages and to learn from and effectively communicate with professionals in the field who were knowledgeable and bilingual and who understood their culture. Many parents also noted that the experience served to clarify their misconceptions, change negative or unrealistic attitudes and expectations, and help them acquire increased understanding of their children's condition and developmental needs. This enabled them to further acquire greater confidence and specific skills in promoting their children's development in various areas. Parents similarly gained a sense of improved self-reliance and personal advocacy through increased awareness of their basic rights and of specific community resources and methods of accessing them; a great many immigrant parents learned of such resources and their entitlements for the very first time.

As they developed self-help skills in obtaining needed services, many parents were often directly assisted by the parent trainers who expedited referrals for a variety of services and programs, transported and accompanied parents to various agencies, translated materials and served as interpreters for parents, and offered personal advice and informal counseling and support. While providing such assistance, the parent trainers demonstrated a high level of sensitivity and increasing self-confidence in relating to both parents and professionals. This growth was also manifested in their increasingly sophisticated group organization and facilitation skills.

The service providers further empowered their respective parent trainer partners by recognizing their primary leadership roles and providing needed support. Throughout this process, many service providers indicated that they developed greater awareness of and sensitivity to the distinct cultural orientations, needs, and personal difficulties of recent immigrant families who have children with disabilities. They also demonstrated increasing enthusiasm and commitment to raising the consciousness of fellow professionals (both within their own agencies and in the community) with regard to the value of MTOT Project parent groups. They emphasized the importance of treating parents "like people" instead of clients and of advocating the parents' right to access needed services. Many providers were further motivated by the parents' dedication and sustained involvement to actively promote the establishment of longer-term parent training programs and support groups.

Project impact

The MTOT Project teams affiliated with the various project sites engaged in a transitional planning process during the final months of formal program support. Efforts were thus directed toward identifying resources and methods of maintaining the established MTOT Project community-based programs. Parent-participants were highly motivated and committed to sustaining their involvement, to continuing to meet and enhance their training experiences, and to recruiting additional parents in the community to joint their groups.

A particularly significant development was the subsequent organization of formal parent groups among the various Asian MTOT Project participants. Within 2 years after completion of the project, selected parent trainers had assumed instrumental leadership roles in guiding the establishment and incorporation of parent organizations serving Chinese, Korean, and Vietnamese families with children with disabilities. These organizations have engaged in pioneering efforts to provide mutual support, education and training, and advocacy for their members and respective communities.

While directly supporting such efforts, former MTOT Project staff have continued to participate actively in resource sharing and the development of parent–professional coalitions and communication networks. Corresponding dissemination efforts have been directed toward the distribution of project information and materials and the provision of technical assistance and consultation to numerous agencies, organizations, and parent-training programs throughout the country. Such efforts have served to augment existing limited resources and to prompt parents, advocates, planners, administrators, and providers to address systematically the needs of underserved populations in their respective communities.

FUTURE DIRECTIONS

The clear intent of Public Law 99-457 is to empower families and promote meaningful involvement in early intervention programs for their children with disabilities, which includes family participation in policy making and program design.[7,8] The corresponding need for greater representation of culturally diverse families in relevant leadership roles has been well established. Each of the previously described parent education and training projects served as part of a model training continuum through which parents from various ethnic groups proceeded. Parent leaders subsequently emerged as family advocates and representatives who could serve on appropriate advisory and policy-making bodies. Such leadership development efforts should be intensified to ensure that service delivery systems are increasingly responsive to the needs of culturally diverse populations.

Comprehensive multicultural training for early intervention personnel is also necessary to facilitate effective service delivery and family and professional collaboration at all levels of care. In response to this need, the UAP at Childrens' Hospital Los Angeles has developed the Multicultural Education and Training (MET) Project. Supported through a 3-year federal grant, the MET Project is directed toward developing, implementing, evaluating, and disseminating a model curriculum of comprehensive multicultural education and training. This curriculum specifically addresses the elements of "cultural competence"[9] that include

1. self-awareness and *awareness* of the "dynamics of difference" (including understanding "culture" and its function in human behavior),
2. *knowledge* of culture-specific information pertaining to various ethnic groups, and
3. *skills* necessary to engage in successful cross-cultural interactions with culturally diverse populations.

This project should thus serve to promote the dissemination of multicultural training concepts, values, and methodologies that reinforce the importance of people culture (vs paper culture) and the critical role it plays in serving infants and young children with disabilities and their families.

REFERENCES

1. US Bureau of the Census. *The Hispanic Population in the United States.* Washington, DC: GPO Series P-20, No. 416.
2. Winget P. California resources in special education: Exploding cross-cultural populations prompt reform of educational system. *Special Edge* November 1989;4(3):1.
3. Johnson BH, McGonigel MJ, Kaufmann RK. *Guidelines and Recommended Practices for the Individualized Family Service Plan.* Washington, DC: Association for the Care of Children's Hospital, 1989.
4. Anderson PP, Schrag Fenichel E. *Serving Culturally Diverse Families of Infants and Toddlers with Disabilities.* Washington, DC: National Center for Clinical Infant Programs, 1989.
5. Smith-Davis J, Burke PJ, Noel M. *Personnel to Educate the Handicapped in America: Supply and Demand from a Programmed Viewpoint.* College Park, Md: Institute for the Study of Exceptional Children and Youth, Department of Special Education, University of Maryland, 1984.
6. Ramirez BA, *Specific Provisions of P.L. 99-457 Related to Special Populations.* Reston, Va: The Council for Exceptional Children, 1987.
7. Dunst CJ, Trivette CM, Deal AG. *Enabling and Empowering Families: Principles and Guidelines for Practice.* Cambridge, Mass: Brookline, 1988.
8. Gallagher JJ, Trohanis PL, Clifford, RM. *Policy Implementation of PL 99-457.* Baltimore: Paul H. Brookes, 1989.
9. Cross T. Services to minority populations: What does it mean to be a culturally competent professional? *Focal Point* 1988;2:1–5.

Impact of feeding problems on the parent–infant relationship

Ruth Humphry, PhD, OTR/L
Division of Occupational Therapy
University of North Carolina
Chapel Hill, North Carolina

EATING PROBLEMS during infancy and the associated feeding difficulties for caregivers have been linked with a variety of developmental and medical problems.[1–3] Once feeding problems are identified, they are reported to persist for an extended period of time.[4] The duration of the problem is significantly longer when the infant is developmentally delayed.[5] Although child-focused assessment and treatment procedures are discussed in the literature,[6–10] feeding an infant is a two-person process, and the role of the second person, the caregiver, should be integrated into any discussion of problems.[11] When considering intervention programs for infants with eating problems, the broader implications for other aspects of the child's development and relationship to family function need to be addressed.[12–14]

An infant's difficulty in eating creates problems for parent–child interaction.[1] Clinicians and researchers have observed that some infants with eating problems have mothers who appear withdrawn and that the mothers' interaction with their children may be poor.[4,11] The association between nonorganic failure to thrive and a higher incidence of oral-motor problems[15,16] raises additional concern; the infant's problems in eating could exacerbate poor caregiving practices. This article considers the consequences for the developing parent–infant relationship of feeding problems based on the infant's developmental or medical status.

As the field's understanding of the complex process of development increases, it becomes clearer that one aspect of caregiving cannot be isolated from another. Feeding is a major activity that is repeated several times a day, and it offers the infant and caregiver valuable learning experiences as they coordinate actions to meet the infant's nutritional needs. The experience of parent–infant interaction, which occurs throughout the feeding process, contributes to the developing relationship.

PROBLEMS FOR THE PARENT–INFANT DYAD

The impact of infant eating problems on the parent–infant relationship can be understood using the transactional model of development.[17] Face-to-face interaction is bidirectional[18]; the abilities of both the parent and infant to engage in their respective roles influence where the relationship falls along a continuum. The quality of the relationship can range from positive and growth enhancing for both parent and infant to negative and destructive. An important aspect of the transactional model is that the strengths of one member of the dyad can compensate for difficulty experienced by the other member. As a result, the development of an infant with special needs may be less influenced by biological risk factors when an adult can compensate and provide the modifications during interaction.[17,19]

Inf Young Children 1991; 3(3): 30–38

The infant and parent–infant interaction

Infant development

One important determinant of how a parent and infant interact is the infant's developmental level.[20] An infant's experiences in being fed can promote sensory, motor, and cognitive development as well as offer social learning situations.[13,21] The oral area is an early source of sensory information about objects in the environment. When there is a problem with the infant's eating abilities, the associated learning opportunities may be changed. For example, if feeding becomes regulated by a schedule, the contingency sequence of infant fuss, caregiver response, and infant relief does not occur as often. In addition, the relaxed interaction during or after mealtime can be lost as both partners are fatigued or stressed by the process of getting food into the infant. The range of opportunities lost by infants not able to be fed are reflected in clinical recommendations regarding promoting the development of a child who is tube fed.[22]

The young infant's control over his or her level of arousal is another issue that may affect the parent–infant relationship. Parents of infants with special needs report more problems with state regulation than parents whose infants are developing normally.[5,23] Sucking can be a mechanism to help state organization[24] and is an effective means of relieving distress.[25] Infants with oral-motor problems may be missing an important ability that enhances self-regulation and allows opportunities for interaction with the parent.

A feeding problem also affects the parent–infant relationship by compromising the social interaction abilities of infants. The infant's difficulty taking in food usually represents a symptom of an underlying medical problem or developmental delay. The same condition may concurrently affect the infant's social behaviors, which subsequently influence the developing relationship. Using microanalysis in observational studies, researchers have identified subtle ways infants influence interactive and feeding behaviors of adults.[13,21] Eye gaze, facial expression, and body movements are the basis for many of the interactive skills of the infant.

Oral-motor problems

Since severe oral-motor problems are associated with other difficulties in movement, studies that have examined parent–infant interaction when the infant has motor problems can shed light on the effects of feeding problems. Of particular interest are two studies in which the design included a second group of infants with special needs but no physical handicaps.[20,26] This method allowed the researchers to separate the impact of characteristics of the child's handicapping conditions from the general influence of the infant's special needs status. These studies and another[27] also compared mother–infant dyads containing physically handicapped infants (usually with cerebral palsy) to other mother–infant pairs with normally developing children. Subjects were matched based on mental and/or chronological age.

There is conflicting evidence regarding the effect of an infant's motor problems on the ability to participate during interaction. In one study,[20] infants with cerebral palsy were less responsive than infants with Down syndrome or general developmental delays. Other researchers[26,27] reported no differences in the amount of the infant's interactive behaviors when infants with motor problems were compared to a matched group of infants with mental retardation and no motor problems or another group of infants of the same developmental age. Results suggest the need for further research with care in selecting the coding system used to record interactive behaviors.[28] For example, infants with motor problems may need additional response time or have alternative means of signaling. Parents of children with motor problems may be able to identify cues that researchers traditionally have not used in their coding of interactive behaviors.

A related issue is the responsivity of mothers who care for infants with motor problems. Yoder and Feagan[29] found, in contradiction to suggestions of decreased maternal involvement, that mothers of severely handicapped infants attribute more communication to infant behavior than women whose infants were developing normally. One study[20] of parent–infant interaction reported no differences in maternal responsivity for handicapped or normal babies but found a strong association with the child's level of cognitive functioning regardless of the presence or type of handicapping condition. Hanzlik and Stevenson[26] also reported no difference in positive responsiveness by mothers of children with or without developmental problems.

A significant increase in the frequency of commands used by the mothers when the child has a handicapping condition has been found.[26,27] The increased amount of directiveness appears to be linked with the presence of a handicapping condition rather than motor problems.[26] Mahoney and his colleagues[30] suggest that the mothers of infants with developmental delays may approach interaction with their infants differently. Increased maternal directiveness suggests more emphasis on instruction or teaching the infant than a relaxed social interaction. Additional research is needed to determine if differences in the parent's interactive intent is beneficial to young children with developmental delays. A related research issue is whether the presence of eating problems causes the parent to approach each meal time as another therapy session, thus reducing the social interaction and increasing directiveness.

Physical appearance

The implications of the infant's physical appearance for caregiver–infant interaction also warrants discussion. Difficulty in eating may be associated with a craniofacial abnormality. An increase in the amount of time the mother ignores her toddler with a physical handicap has led some researchers to suggest that the mother gradually withdraws from a child with a visible handicap.[31] Two observational studies[32,33] examined interaction of mothers and their infants with craniofacial deformities and compared them to mother–infant dyads where the infant had no birth defect. The earlier research[32] reported fewer positive interactive behaviors (eg, infant gaze behavior, maternal responsivity) by both the mother and infant when the infant had facial anomalies. The second study[33] similarly found less maternal interaction and warmth when the infant had a facial deformity. Although a small sample size is a limiting feature of the second study, the fact that infants with deformities touched their mothers and smiled less and looked away more than infants without physical deformities raises concern about the parent–infant relationship. The nature of behavioral differences during interaction warrant further study, because parents of infants with facial deformities report more satisfaction in parenting.[33]

These selected observational studies indicate that the parent–infant relationship is an abstract, multifaceted, social bond. As a note of precaution in interpreting observational studies, the potential for observer bias favoring more attractive subjects in coding interaction has recently been suggested.[34] One positive move in research on parent–infant interaction has been an increased use of alternative methodologies.[35] Evidence from several sources should be used to draw conclusions about the developing parent–infant relationship when the infant has special needs.

The parent and parent–infant interaction

To appreciate the consequences of feeding problems on the parent–infant relationship, an understanding of the second member of the dyad involved in feeding the infant is essential. Although most clinicians have a detailed understanding of the infant's developing oral-motor skills necessary for eating, they may not understand how adults acquire parenting skills such as feeding. Yet, when the infant's problems cannot be eliminated, changing parenting practices or family routines becomes a target in early intervention.[36] Reflecting the growing acceptance of a transactional model of development, a number of studies[35,37] have included variables related to the parent, fueling a growing appreciation of the factors that contribute to individual parenting differences.

Adult development

Feeding, part of a complex process of caregiving, offers opportunities for the development of the adult's caregiver role. When an infant is born, the parent must organize a new self-concept as parent for that particular child.[38] Feeding the infant is a very tangible part of the nurturing process, and weight gain is often viewed as evidence of success in the parenting role. Observation of the child's growth promotes the adult's psychosocial development. Presumed failure in the caregiver role in the case of an infant who does not gain weight may have an impact on the adult's developing concept of self as parent.

Caregiving behaviors are not automatic but are acquired as part of a developmental process. A parent's role definition of "good parenting" is shaped by his or her experiences as a child.[37] A woman's mental image of her relationship with her child emerges before the infant is born and will mediate how she interacts with her infant.[39] This internal working model appears to be based, in part, on how the parent was parented. For example, Crowell and Feldman[40] used mothers' memories of their relationships with their mothers to classify the quality of past mother–child attachment.[40] The researchers then examined the quality of the infant's attachment to the mother and found an association with the quality of the woman's past relationships. A parent who was nurtured as a child anticipates caregiving behaviors that are responsive to his or her child's needs. Each parent's internal model of parent–infant relationship influences how that parent interacts with a difficult-to-feed infant.

Education in caregiving skills

In addition to childhood memories of being parented, new parents search for resources to obtain specific knowledge and skills for feeding. The parent's present social and cultural situation influences where the adult turns to learn more about parenting or child development.[41] For example, middle-class mothers are more likely to turn to professionals for advice.[42] In examining feeding practices of new mothers, McLorg and Bryant[43] describe a social network of influences. The different subcultures of the women in the study were related to whether the mother's own mother or the child's physician were named as primary sources of advice. Social group status also influenced the extent to which the parent followed advice about feeding the infant. Recognition of the sources of influence on parenting practices is important. If the professional assumes that he or she is the primary source of information on feeding infants, the parent may be viewed as noncompliant[44] rather than simply integrating one additional source with the many others and evolving his or her individual parenting style.

Increased appreciation of parents as thinking partners has led to studies regarding what parents know about development and the extent to which their beliefs shape parenting behavior.[45] Realistic expectations can influence the parent's satisfaction with the child's behaviors. Parents, regardless of previous experiences with children, have been judged not to be very accurate about developmental milestones.[46] However, another study[41] suggests that when the milestone has special cultural meaning, the expectations were accurate. When examining what parents know about development, an important issue for further study is what parents view as relevant developmental changes. For most parents, the infant's transition to new food textures may be viewed as automatic. The infant who is developing normally may initiate a transition in feeding by reaching for food the adult is eating or grabbing at the spoon when being fed. The child with physical problems may not give the parents the same cues. Until the child has eating problems, the parent may not seek out or value information on alternative feeding practices or be aware of the developmental progression to new foods.

Personality traits

An additional source of influence on how a parent responds to an infant is the adult's emotional or psychological status.[37] Although there are many different types of personality traits of potential interest, depression has been studied extensively in the past few years. Postpartum depression has recently been reviewed in this journal.[47] Research on depression is of particular interest to clinicians if the parent reacts to difficulty in feeding the infant by becoming withdrawn. The infant develops an internal model of relationships based on interaction with his or her parent.[39] Infants of depressed women were found to have depressed interaction with other adults as well as with their mothers.[48] Related to the potential impact of feeding problems on the parent's self-concept, parental depression warrants continued research effort and clinical attention.

Another personality trait that has received attention in the literature is internal or external locus of control.[49] The belief that one is able to affect a life situation is considered a personality trait that varies among individuals. The potential impact of an adult's sense of control on parenting suggests care in interpretation of what a parent says. One study[50] found that a mistaken sense of control over infant crying was associated with mothers who were more depressed and had poorer infant attachment. Another study[51] found that when women expressed the belief that their behavior may have contributed to birth complications, the women had better adjustment to later caregiving problems and were more responsible to their infants' needs. In some situations, "self-blame" may reflect a sense of control, which extends to the parent's feeling the ability to influence the child's developmental outcome. When dealing with an infant that is difficult to feed, a parent with an internal sense of control may recognize the problem and seek out resources. At other times, erroneous illusion of control may be a form of denial that the situation is beyond the individual's influence. This false sense of influence may be a maladaptive coping mechanism[50] and, in the case of a difficult-to-feed child, may make the parent less responsive to the child's cues for changes in the feeding process or open to professional suggestions.

INTERVENTION STRATEGIES

Experiences with feeding influence the developmental progress of the parent and infant. Interactive behaviors of the dyad may be directly or indirectly affected by characteristics of the underlying problem in the infant associated with the eating dysfunction. Research on individual differences among parents suggests different ways a parent might react to difficulty in feeding the infant. A parent–infant relationship does not evolve in a vacuum, and the impact of the family system on the parent–infant subsystem and the reciprocal impact of the dyad on general family function should be recognized. Early intervention or medical services often become part of the relationship's ecological picture when the child has problems gaining weight. Traditional intervention strategies for infants with eating problems have been to modify the feeding process to compensate for the infant's dysfunction.[6,7]

A holistic approach is necessary to ameliorate feeding problems. Clinical observations[2,52] suggest that parents may become consumed with feeding if the child has a history of eating problems or may misinterpret the infant's behavior during feeding and contribute to the problem. If feeding issues compromise the general quality of the parent–infant relationship, the child may be at risk for a less-than-optimal long-term outcome even when nutritional status is improved.

Assessment

The clinician must begin by understanding the parent's perception of the infant's problem.[53] Seligman and Darling[54] examined the meaning of a developmental disability and revealed that there is a wide range of potential reactions based on the parent's subculture's perspective of birth defect. The foundation of the intervention plan for feeding problems should include a family assessment.[55,56] The meaning of the child's behaviors around mealtime needs to be explored with the parents. The caregiver should also identify the parents' other sources of advice on parenting practices. Professional recommendations consistent with the social network that influences feeding practices will increase the probability of family application. The history of the parent's past may include information related to the parent–infant relationship and feeding practices. The parent's right to privacy should be respected, though. Information about the parent's own history or child-rearing attitudes may emerge over time, adding to the early interventionist's understanding of the best way to adapt recommendations. A key to successful assessment is allowing time to gather information, make home visits, and establish a working relationship with families.

Implementation

Feeding difficulties may be a source of parent–professional stress. The health implications of failure to thrive may motivate the professional to identify needed changes in the parent's feeding practices, which may not be implemented. Parenting is influenced by a number of factors, and professional input may not be weighted as heavily as advice from others in the parent's social network. In addition, professionals use knowledge about child development to guide intervention strategies. Literature suggests that what a parent knows about development is only one source of influence on parenting, and knowledge has only a weak relationship with behavior.[45] As a result, early interventionists who assume that telling parents about feeding and nutrition is sufficient to change parenting practices may become frustrated. At times, professionals may feel the parent is contributing to the child's failure to gain weight. Rather than concentrating solely on family compliance, an understanding of factors that influence implementation is an important area for research.[44]

In addition, clinicians should exercise caution when suggesting that if the parent adopts new feeding practices, the child's nutritional status will automatically improve. Treatment of oral-motor dysfunction is still evolving, and efficacy has not been established.[14] Even when gastrostomy feeding is initiated, the child may still not gain the expected weight.[57] Parents may begin to doubt professional advice if adoption of feeding suggestions does not lead to infant weight gain.

Teamwork of parents and professionals is needed in all aspects of early intervention, particularly in feeding. Studies[51,58] have demonstrated that intervention programs may only be effective if the parent feels a need to participate. Feeding a child may take several hours a day,[59] and the parents may decide that they have found the way that is best for overall family function. Therapeutic suggestions need to be evaluated in light of how much time any intervention will take and its impact on other aspects of parent–infant interaction.[60] Strategies that enhance the parent's sense of control over some aspect of the infant's condition will be important.

Feeding programs that focus exclusively on getting the food into the child deal with only part of the problem. Alternatives to a child-focused "infant stimulation" approach and more emphasis on parent–infant interaction have been proposed.[61–64] Positive developmental outcomes have been found when the parent is provided with information about child development rather than behavior management skills[65] and is engaged in a problem-solving approach.[61] Intervention programs that specifically emphasize supporting optimal parent–infant interaction have been successful in reducing the amount of physical directiveness[66] and increasing the responsiveness of the parent.[62]

• • •

Application of the transactional model suggests intervention strategies that promote parent–infant interaction. A strong parent–infant relationship has potential for maximal compensation for medical and developmental problems that result in eating problems. How relationship-focused programs are carried out with medically fragile or severely involved infants who are difficult to feed needs further clarification and research. A further step will be to avoid an exclusive focus on the mechanical process of getting nutrients into the child and instead to recognize the importance of the feeding process in the parent–infant relationship.

REFERENCES

1. Brizee LS, Sophos CM, McLaughlin JF. Nutrition issues in developmental disabilities. *Inf Young Children.* 1990;2:10–21.
2. Puntis JWL, Ritson DG, Holden CE, Buick RG. Growth and feeding problems after repair of oesophageal atresia. *Arch Dis Child.* 1990;65:84–88.
3. Singer LT, Wood R, Lambert S. Developmental follow-up of long-term infant tracheostomy: A preliminary report. *Dev Behav Pediatr.* 1985;6:132–136.
4. Dahl M, Sundelin C. Early feeding problems in an affluent society. *Acta Paediatr Scand.* 1986;75:370–379.
5. Blackman JA, Cobb LS. A comparison of parents' perceptions of common behavior problems in developmentally at-risk and normal children. *Child Health Care.* 1989;18:108–113.
6. Alexander R. Oral-motor treatment for infants and young children with cerebral palsy. *Semi Speech Lang.* 1987;8:87–100.
7. Copeland ME, Kimmel JR. *Evaluation and Management of Infants and Young Children with Developmental Disabilities.* Baltimore, Md: Paul H. Brookes; 1989.
8. Leaf JP, Gisel EG. Neonatal sucking behavior: A quick method of evaluation through structured visual observation. *Phys Occup Ther Pediatr.* 1986;6:27–37.
9. McBride MC, Danner SC. Sucking disorders in neurologically impaired infants: Assessment and facilitation of breast feeding. *Clin Perinatol.* 1987;14:109–130.
10. Sheppard JJ. Assessment of oral motor behaviors in cerebral palsy. *Semin Speech Lang.* 1987;8:57–70.
11. Woolston JL. Eating disorders in infancy and early childhood. *J Am Acad Child Psychiatry.* 1983;22:114–121.
12. Bax M. Eating is important. *Dev Med Child Neurol.* 1989;31:285–286.
13. Humphry R. Feeding problems and the mother–infant relationship. In: Pehoski C, ed. *Problems with Eating.* Rockville, Md: American Occupational Therapy Association; 1987.
14. Ottenbacher K, Bundy A, Short MA. The development and treatment of oral-motor dysfunction: A review of clinical research. *Phys Occup Ther Pediatr.* 1983;3:1–13.
15. Heptinstall E, Puckering C, Skuse D, Start K, Zur-Szpiro S, Dowdney L. Nutrition and mealtime behavior in families of growth retarded children. *Hum Nutr Appl Nutr.* 1987;41A:390–402.
16. Mathisen B, Skuse D, Wolke, D, Reilly S. Oral-motor dysfunction and failure to thrive among inner-city infants. *Dev Med Child Neurol.* 1989;31:293–302.
17. Sameroff AJ, Chandler MJ. Reproductive risk and the continuum of caretaking causality. In: Horowitz FD, Heatherington M, Scarr-Salapatek S, Siegel G, eds. *Review of Child Development Research.* Chicago, Ill: University of Chicago Press; 1975;4.
18. Cohn JF, Tronick EZ. Mother–infant face-to-face interaction: Influence is bidirectional and unrelated to periodic cycles in either partner's behavior. *Dev Psychol.* 1988;24:386–392.
19. Aylward GP. Environmental influences on the developmental outcome of children at risk. *Inf Young Children.* 1990;2:1–9.
20. Brooks-Gunn J, Lewis M. Maternal responsivity in the interaction with handicapped infants. *Child Dev.* 1984;55:782–793.
21. Stevenson MB, Roach MA, Ver Hoeve JN, Leavitt LA. Rhythms in the dialogue of infant feeding: Preterm and term infants. *Inf Behav Dev.* 1990;13:51–70.

22. Wink DM. The physical and emotional care of infants with gastrostomy tubes. *Issues Compr Pediatr Nurs.* 1983;6:195–203.
23. Humphry R. When an infant has a feeding problem. *Occup Ther J Res.* In press.
24. Oetter P. *Manual.* Hugo, Minn: PDP Products. In press.
25. Campos RG. Soothing pain-elicited distress in infants with swaddling and pacifiers. *Child Dev.* 1989;60:781–792.
26. Hanzlik JR, Stevenson MB. Interaction of mothers with their infants who are mentally retarded, retarded with cerebral palsy or nonretarded. *Am J Ment Defic.* 1986;90:513–520.
27. Barrera ME, Vella DM. Disabled and nondisabled infants' interaction with their mothers. *Am J Occup Ther.* 1987;41:168–172.
28. Hanzlik JR. Interactions between mothers and their infants with developmental disabilities: Analysis and review. *Phys Occup Ther Pediatr.* 1989;9:33–48.
29. Yoder PJ, Feagan L. Mothers' attribution of communication to prelinguistic behavior of developmentally delayed and mentally retarded infants. *Am J Ment Retardation.* 1988;93:36–43.
30. Mahoney G, Fors S, Wood S. Maternal directive behavior revisited. *Am J Mental Retardation* 1990;94:398–407.
31. Wasserman BA, Allen R. Maternal withdrawal from handicapped toddlers. *Child Psychol Psychiatr.* 1985;26:381–387.
32. Field TM, Vega-Lahr N. Early interactions between infants with cranio-facial anomalies and their mothers. *Inf Behav Dev.* 1984;7:527–530.
33. Barden RC, Ford ME, Jensen AG, Roger-Salyer M, Salyer KE. Effects of cranio-facial deformity in infancy on the quality of mother–infant interaction. *Child Dev.* 1989;60:819–824.
34. Ritter JM, Laglois JH. The role of physical attractiveness in the observation of adult–child interactions: Eye of the beholder or behavioral reality? *Dev Psychol.* 1988;24:254–263.
35. Parke RD, Tinsley BJ. Family interaction in infancy. In: Osofsky JD, ed. *Handbook of Infant Development.* New York, NY: Wiley; 1987.
36. Fiese BH, Sameroff AJ. Family context in pediatric psychology: A transactional perspective. *J Pediatr Psychol.* 1989;14:293–314.
37. Belsky J. The determinants of parenting: A process model. *Child Dev.* 1984;55:83–96.
38. Partridge SE. The parental self-concept: A theoretical exploration and practical application. *Am J Orthopsychiatry.* 1988;58:281–287.
39. Zeanah CH, Anders TF. Subjectivity in parent–infant relationship: A discussion of internal working models. *Inf Ment Health J.* 1987;8:237–250.
40. Crowell JA, Feldman SS. Mothers' internal models of relationships and children's behavior and developmental status: A study of mother–child interaction. *Child Dev.* 1988;59:1273–1285.
41. Hopkins B, Westra T. Maternal expectations of their infants' development: Some cultural differences. *Dev Med Child Neurol.* 1989;31:384–390.
42. While AE. Early infant feeding practice: Socioeconomic factors and health visiting support. *Child Health Care.* 1989;15:129–136.
43. McLorg PA, Bryant CA. Influence of social network members and health care professionals on infant feeding practices of economically disadvantaged mothers. *Med Anthropology.* 1989;10: 265–278.
44. Trostle JA. Medical compliance as an ideology. *Soc Sci Med.* 1988;27:1299–1308.
45. Miller SA. Parents' beliefs about children's cognitive development. *Child Dev.* 1988;59:259–285.

46. Reiss J. Child-rearing expectations and developmental knowledge according to maternal age and parity. *Inf Ment Health J.* 1988;9:287–304.
47. Short-DeGraph MA, Healey SM. Postpartum depression related to care for the child with special needs. *Inf Young Children.* 1989;2:24–36.
48. Field T, Healy B, Goldstein S, et al. Infants of depressed mothers show "depressed" behavior even with nondepressed adults. *Child Dev.* 1988;59:1569–1579.
49. Friedrich WN, Cohen DS, Wilturner LT. Specific beliefs and moderator variables in maternal coping with mental retardation. *Child Health Care.* 1988;17:40–44.
50. Donovan WL, Leavitt LA. Maternal self-efficacy and infant attachment: Integrating physiology, perceptions and behaviors. *Child Dev.* 1989;60:460–472.
51. Affleck G, Tennen H, Rowe J, Roscher B, Walker L. Effects of formal support on mother's adaptation to the hospital-to-home transition of high risk infants: The benefits and costs to helping. *Child Dev.* 1989;60:488–501.
52. Cramer BG. Objective and subjective aspects of parent–infant relations: An attempt at correlation between infant studies and clinical work. In: Osofsky JD, ed. *Handbook of Infant Development.* 2nd ed. New York, NY: Wiley; 1987.
53. Hodapp RM. The role of maternal emotions and perceptions in interactions with young handicapped children. In: Marfo K, ed. *Parent–Child Interaction and Developmental Disabilities.* New York, NY: Praeger; 1988.
54. Seligman M, Darling R. *Ordinary Families, Special Children.* New York, NY: Guilford Press; 1989.
55. Bailey DB, Simeonsson RJ, eds. *Family Assessment in Early Intervention.* Columbus, OH, Merrill Publishing Company; 1988.
56. Turnbull AP, Turnbull HR. *Families, Professionals and Exceptionality.* Columbus, Ohio: Charles E. Merrill; 1986.
57. Rempel GR, Colwell SO, Nelson RP. Growth in children with cerebral palsy fed via gastrostomy. *Pediatrics.* 1988;82:857–862.
58. Belsky J. A tale of two variances: Between and within. *Child Dev.* 1986;57:1301–1305.
59. Jones PM. Feeding disorders in children with multiple handicaps. *Dev Med Child Neurol.* 1989;31:398–406.
60. Morris S. Therapy for the child with cerebral palsy: Interacting frameworks. *Semin Speech Lang.* 1987;8:71–86.
61. Barrera M, Rosenbaum P. The transactional model of early home intervention. *Inf Ment Health J.* 1986;7:112–131.
62. Mahoney G, Powell A. Modifying parent–child interaction: Enhancing the development of handicapped children. *J Spec Educ.* 1988;22:82–96.
63. Rauh VA, Achenbach TM, Nurcombe B, Howell CT, Teti DM. Minimizing adverse effects of low birthweight: Four-year results of early intervention program. *Child Dev.* 1988;59:544.
64. Bromwich RM. The interaction approach to early intervention. *Inf Ment Health J.* 1990;11:66–79.
65. Moxley-Heagert L, Servin LA. Developmental education for parents of delayed infants: Effects on parental motivation and children's development. *Child Dev.* 1983;54:1324–1331.
66. Hanzlik JR. The effect of intervention on the free-play experience for mothers and their infants with developmental delay and cerebral palsy. *Phys Occup Ther Pediatr.* 1989;9:33–51.

Fathers: Myth, reality, and Public Law 99-457

Joyce W. Sparling, PhD, PT, OT
Assistant Professor
Project Director, Maternal and Child Health Training Grant

Robert G. Berger, MD
Director, Outpatient Medicine

Michael E. Biller
Division of Physical Therapy
School of Medicine
University of North Carolina
Chapel Hill, North Carolina

THE TERM "family" is not synonymous with "mother," yet mothers consistently have been the focus of family intervention related to children with or at risk of chronic of disabling conditions.[1] Even though there has been a dramatic increase in research related to fathering and program development in the last 15 to 20 years, the lack of inclusion of fathers in special programming persists. This fact may be due to a historical characterization of fathers as uninvolved in the development and education of their special children.

To describe the evolution of this characterization, the literature on the historical and cultural role of the father will be reviewed. This information will be related to federal legislation supporting the education of children 0 to 21 years of age[2] and to fathers' interaction with their special children. Based on a review of current literature on special children and their fathers and on personal and professional experience with special children, the authors will suggest eight factors critical to family-centered intervention that includes fathers. Three questions will guide this review:

1. Do fathers want to be involved in decision-making and intervention?
2. Do educational personnel need to attend to a variety of paternal perspectives and be responsible for locating, scheduling, and otherwise involving fathers in the assessment and planning for the young child?
3. If father participation is wanted, what approach best facilitates this involvement?

In addressing these questions, it is useful to have an awareness of the changing statistics related to fathers. In 1960, 75% of all families were of the nuclear type (ie, households with husbands and wives), with a decrease to 55% projected for 1990.[3] In addition, two thirds of all types of families were estimated to be without children. Of the families with children, two thirds were projected to include primary or secondary caretaking fathers living in married couple households and primary caretaking fathers living as single parents. Statistics for ethnic groups[4] vary even more, with 53% of black children (compared with 17% of children of other ethnic groups) living in single-parent families. These figures suggest a di-

This work was supported in part by Maternal and Child Health Grant no. 149 and The Carolina Institute for Research on Infant Personnel Preparation Grant no. G0087C3064.

Inf Young Children 1992; 4(3): 9–19

minished role of the nuclear family in American society, a decrease in the number of fathers living within the family, and an increase in primary caretaking fathers.

Changing family structure and its inevitable effect on parental availability is of particular concern in relation to special needs children. With more than 12.65 million children experiencing health problems[5] and authorization pending on adequate funds to address their needs, enactment of Public Law 99-457 is admirable but overwhelming in its challenge. To address family aspects of this challenge, the working definition of families will have to be extended beyond mothers. Because the support of fathers as well as mothers may be essential to the successful implementation of PL 99-457, greater knowledge is needed of fathers' interests, skills, and roles.

HISTORICAL DEFINITION OF THE FATHER

The social role of the father has changed dramatically in the past 100 years. Changes in male roles have been linked inextricably to changes in female roles and to multiple war efforts. At the turn of the century, men were characterized as Victorian omnipotent patriarchs in control of the social as well as financial fortunes of their families. With the advent of war, men became coworkers of wartime work force women. As women left the home and entered the work force, changes occurred in the established equilibrium of the family[6] and modified women's expectations of the father within the family.

With these new expectations of fathers, and in conflict with them, was an entrenched societal view of mothers as the prototypical nurturers and fathers as the prototypical adventurers. Women were the competent caretakers, experienced in all matters related to the child. Men were the inexperienced caretakers who had to learn the competencies of child care. This lack of experience, often encouraged by women, was basic to the establishment of the myth of the "derelict dad."

In the 1960s and 1970s there was an increased interest in and study of the role of the father. Although much of this literature has been based on low-risk populations, the recognition of "normal" paternal parenting attitudes and skills has set the stage for investigations of the unique characteristics of fathers interacting with their special needs children. In the 1960s traditional perspectives of the generic father were modified, fostering a view of the father as "the bridge to the vast world outside."[8] The father-child relationship was interpreted as "the model for many subsequent social relations and involvements."[8] The literature of the 1980s provided further support for this view. Fathers were described as interested in the care of their children,[9,10] although they were not spending as much time as mothers with their children.[11] During this same period, the role of fathers was extended, with father influence being initiated in pregnancy[12,13] and continuing well beyond the early years of the child's development.[14] Further research suggested that paternal interactions with their children appeared to vary with different settings[15] and with children of different characteristics, such as gender[16,17] and maturity at birth.[18] Fathers' interaction came to be characterized as less verbal but more vigorous, physical, and play oriented[19–22] than that of mothers.

Recognizing the uniqueness of paternal behavior in interaction was preliminary to accepting the importance of the male influence on the developing child. The thesis that fathers present different and developmentally appropriate challenges to their children has been supported in a number of recent investigations. For example, one study[23] showed that in communicating with their children, fathers requested clarifications of their childs' comments and often did not acknowledge their children's responses, with these behaviors facilitating the children's language development.

In addition to the uniqueness of men's interaction with children, there appears to be a discrepancy in the literature between expected and actual amount of paternal interaction. Several studies[24,25] suggested that fathers spent 15 to 25 minutes a day interacting with their infant. More recent reports describe fathers as being available to their infants 2¾ hours per weekday, with 45 to 50 minutes of that time spent in actual interaction.[11] The fathers in this study performed one caretaking activity per day and took care of the infant by themselves once in 10 days. Results of this study suggested that fathers who spend more time with their infants attribute greater cognitive competence to them and therefore create a mutually reinforcing interaction with their children. This study was conducted in Israel and suggests that there is a culture of fathers that transcends national boundaries.

CULTURAL DEFINITION OF THE FATHER

Consistent with the concept of men as adventurers is the idea that "men's cultural heritage and biophysical endowment ill equip them to participate in the networks of interpersonal intimacy."[26] This sort of emphasis on gender differences has been applied directly to parental roles, as noted in statements such as, "Any society that may have attempted to equilibrate the parental roles did not compete effectively against societies stressing the mother role and has quietly disappeared with no trace."[27(p156)]

To determine whether there were generic characteristics distancing fathers from their children, Mackey conducted extensive cross-cultural studies with fathers.[28] He observed 49,000 adults and children in 18 cultures across five continents in the late 1970s and early 1980s and concluded that given a "reasonably stable environment . . . men in a tribe or community will gravitate toward their children and nurture, cuddle, and play with them. . . . They will love their children because they are built to love them."[28(pp 176,177)] He summarized his results by stating that "the myth of the derelict dad"[28(p142)] no longer exists. Instead, fathers as well as children need interaction. The way in which this interaction is implemented is dependent on the unique characteristics of the individuals involved. Pruett's work[29] with primary care fathers and their working spouses supports this thesis and suggests that freedom in role choice may be a critical family issue in contrast to gender determination of roles.

Thus it may be that fathers generally want to facilitate the education of their children, but under situations of stress that create an unstable family environment (eg, poverty, racial discrimination, employment and social competition, or child impairment), paternal participation in the family and child education may be limited and intervention may need to be culture specific. Research on cultural traditions and expectations may foster a deeper understanding of special children and their families[30–32] and help interventionists more effectively meet the demands of the new legislation.

CURRENT FEDERAL LEGISLATION

Public Law 99-457, The Education of the Handicapped Act Amendments of 1986,[2] is a continuation of federal policy initiated by PL 99-142, which ensured appropriate education for all children 5 to 21 years of age and a state discretionary clause providing education for all children 3 to 5 years of age. Title I of PL 99-457 extends this initiative to children from birth through 2 years of age. The Part H amendment is based on four "findings" that support an "urgent and substantial need" to (1) facilitate development and decrease delays in handicapped infants and toddlers, (2) to decrease school-age educational costs, (3) to foster "the potential for independent living" and (4) to help families "meet the special needs" of their children. To meet these needs, the amendment establishes a new state grant program to benefit children who have delayed development, have a condition that may result in a delay, or are at risk for delay. Although the states have latitude in the development of their programs, requirements include multidisciplinary assessment, case management, and an Individualized Family Service Plan (IFSP).

The IFSP is one of the most challenging components of the Part H amendment. Its stipulations are described in Section 677 of the amendment and are shown in Table 1. They clearly indicate that the family as well as the child is the focus of the IFSP process. Although the case manager no doubt involves the family in transitions in school placement, that activity is not clearly enumerated in the regulations.

The process of meeting these stipulations includes consultation with all individuals involved in the education of the child: the parents as well as the teachers who provide learning opportunities and the disciplinary representatives who support the special needs of the child and those of the family relative to the child. The challenge for this multidisciplinary team is to produce an intervention plan for the child that is consistent with goals prioritized by the family.

Table 1. "Multidisciplinary" team stipulations for meeting IFSP requirements for family and special child

Family	*Child*
Determine "strengths and needs"	Determine present level of development
Select major outcomes expected	Select major outcomes expected
Identify specific services including starting dates and duration	Identify specific services including starting dates and duration
Designate case manager	Designate a case manager
	Prepare for transition to new school setting

For those fathers who want to become involved with the team, three problems related to the regulations exist: (1) the use of the singular term, "parent or guardian," rather than the plural, "parents"; (2) the kind of team designated to develop the IFSP; and (3) professional lack of knowledge about families. These problems are fundamental to all involvement, yet are particularly evident for any minority group such as fathers.

First, the designation of "parent" rather than "parents," stated in Section 677, assumes that as long as one parent or guardian is involved on the team, family views are represented. In a recent analysis of completed IFSPs,[33] only 2% of the reviewed IFSP goals related specifically to the father. In this report, the goal for the father was "Dad will learn to simplify activities that he enjoys so child can participate." It would appear that fathers are not only inadequately represented in IFSP goals, but few teams have identified the inclusion of the father as a priority.

To determine the reason for this apparent noninvolvement of fathers, a survey was conducted of 31 public school physical therapists attending a statewide continuing education conference (Sparling JW, unpublished results, November 1990). Ninety-four percent of the therapists believed that fathers could have a "marked influence on child development," and 71% tried to include them in the Individual Education Program (IEP/IFSP) process. Only 33%, however, communicated regularly with fathers living with their children, and only 7% communicated with fathers living in a different home than their children. The variety of reasons given by these therapists for and against father involvement are shown in Table 2.

The second problem for fathers relates to the composition and goals of the intervention team itself. There are three types of teams described in the intervention literature.[34] *Multidisciplinary* refers to disciplines acting independently, whereas *interdisciplinary* describes active interaction among disciplines, and *transdisciplinary* refers to members sharing aspects of each other's responsibilities. The term *multidisciplinary* is used to describe teams within PL 99-457. In Report 99-860 from the Committee on Education and Labor,[35] which provided

Table 2. Reasons for and against including fathers in their child's educational process

Against	*For*
Therapist's time limited because of large caseload (range, 7–60)	Father provides less stressful intervention than mother (ie, ability to facilitate play with child)
Father's lack of interest and inaccessibility	Father may lighten mother's child responsibilities (eg, provide transportation)
Father's lack of knowledge of child and caregiving	Father can develop and repair child's equipment
Father's lack of time	Father can act as role model
Father's rejection of child's need for special care and instruction	Father can participate in exercise regimen

consultation in developing the amendment, the more appropriate term *interdisciplinary,* rather than multidisciplinary, was used to describe teams. In light of the lack of interaction that is characteristic of multidisciplinary teams, the potential for these teams to achieve IFSP goals is in question. It also may be difficult for a father to participate vigorously on a multidisciplinary team that traditionally espouses disciplinary rather than child/family goals. For example, a therapist may suggest a detailed home program specifying paternal involvement, but the father who is working two jobs neither understands nor values the program or is too exhausted to participate in it.

The third potential problem of the amendment in relation to fathers is the professional lack of knowledge of fathers' unique interests, skills, and schedules. In recent surveys by special educators, physical therapists, speech and language pathologists, occupational therapists, and physicians, the lack of these professionals' knowledge of family structure functions and needs has been clearly identified.[36–40] Professionals to date have been concerned with the IFSP process,[41,42] but little has been written about the actual way in which professionals acquire parent information related to children's goals. The few skills that have been designated by some interventionists as critical in interacting with parents include interviewing and observation.[43–45] The ability to lead group discussions with parents and team members[46] and to coordinate team efforts are additional skills needed in interacting with fathers. Skills such as these are now being identified for instruction at the preservice and in-service levels,[47] and curricula are being modified (Sparling JW, unpublished data, 1991).

FATHERS AND THEIR SPECIAL NEEDS CHILDREN

Public Law 99-457 defines special children as those who are developmentally delayed, have a condition that may result in a delay, or are at risk for delay. Early studies of fathers and their special children were mainly concerned with children already delayed, describing the negative effects of child impairment on fathers in terms of low self-esteem, acceptance of their children, and depression.[48] More recent research has disentangled the results of earlier studies, suggesting that fathers of special children, like other fathers, are not all depressed but vary in their state according to a multitude of factors. For example, Patterson, McCubbin, and Warwick[49] reported that fathers' maintenance of self-esteem, psychological stability, and social support were significantly associated with their child's health status (eg, weight gain and improved pulmonary function). Other studies have supported the effect of child status on the father. In a sample of 148 parents, Ferrari[50] showed that fathers of chronically ill children perceived significantly less social support than did the fathers of children with no identified illness. Frey, Fewell, and Vadasy[51] studied 48 parents and their special needs children, 60% of whom had Down syndrome. The child's standardized communication skill score predicted the father's and mother's adjustment to their child at 1 year, whereas paternal adjustment to his child at 1 year predicted the mother's adjustment at 3 years. In addition to the long-term effect of child status on fathers, this study suggests the potential influence of paternal attitudes toward the child on other family members.

Much of the contemporary research addresses infants who have a condition that may result in a delayed development or are at risk of delay. Work with children who had cystic fibrosis or congenital heart disease[52] and were at risk for delay found that fathers were sensitive to the children's condition, but these conditions had less influence on their daily lives than on the mothers' lives. Fathers were less attached to their infants than were mothers, while reporting less stress than mothers in terms of depression, role restrictions, personal health, and marital problems. These results suggest that fathers may see the handicap in more instrumental ways, whereas mothers interpret it more expressively. Socioeconomic status and child age, however, may be critical variables in our understanding of these results. In a study of relatively affluent parents of Down syndrome children,[53] 83% of the fathers described their adjustment to their children as a slow and steady positive process starting at the time of diagnosis. This adjustment contrasted with the fluctuating, crisis-oriented adjustment of their spouses. These results suggest that fathers appear to benefit from early knowledge of their child's impairment, which may lead to more interactive experiences with the child and greater confidence in their child's competencies, in their paternal roles, and in the father-child relationship.

Children at risk for delay characteristically include premature infants and children from inadequate living environments. In studies related to these children, fathers' employment has been a critical variable, for employment status often determines the availability of the father to the child and simultaneously provides relief from the strain that the child's risk status creates. In addition, work demands on fathers of young children may be greater than demands placed on them after their careers have been established. In a study of 50 preterm infants,[54] frequency of father hospital visits (ie, availability of father to child) showed a significant positive relationship to child weight gain, father's perceptions of the infant, and paternal behaviors in interaction at hospital discharge and at 8 and 18 months. Although paternal availability to the child is important, so, too, is the opportunity for fathers to distance themselves from the strain of child care. In another study[55] of very low birth weight (VLBW) infants, the length of hospitalization of the preterm children did not negatively affect fathers' behaviors as it did mothers' behaviors. The authors suggested that paternal employment supported the fathers' adaptation.

With the increase in two-worker families, employment status and the availability of fathers and mothers for children has become a dominant issue. A positive outcome of "the shared parenting family"[56] may be the potential increase in availability of fathers for interaction with their children. Although this exciting potential may exist, paternal choice related to involvement also needs to exist.[57]

In addition to premature children, there is an increased risk for developmental delay in children of adolescents, many of whom live in conditions of low financial and psychosocial support. Adolescent mothers have reported significantly less paternal involvement with their children than a comparison group of adult mothers.[58] In addition, 43% of second-time adolescent mothers reported the same father for both pregnancies, compared with 84% of second-time adult mothers reporting the same father.[59] In a follow-up of adolescent mothers and their 8-month-old infants,[60] the mother's satisfaction with life was significantly related to her social support. The adolescent mothers' parenting behaviors were associated with their perceptions of current partner support, not the support of their biologic families, although 75% of the teens were not living with the biologic father (40% had new boyfriends; 13% had male relatives providing support; 22% had no male support). Differences in perceptions of social support suggest the need for interventionists to determine individual paternal perceptions about, as well as knowledge of, their special children.

THE FATHER AND PL 99-457: INTERVENTION

The involvement of the father in the education of his special child apparently is based on the father's availability and his perception of his child's competency.[11] Programs that have been responsive to these two factors have met with paternal participation that has benefited both the child and the father. Programs and projects that seem to support fathers the most include four major components: (1) father involvement in program planning; (2) convenience in program scheduling (ie, weekday evenings, Saturdays); (3) projects that increase the father's knowledge base related to his child; and (4) opportunities for the father to enjoy activities with his child. These components will be described briefly as interpreted by the following four projects: the Seattle Extended Family Program (SEFAM), the Families and Work Institute's Fatherhood Project, Revelj's physical therapy program, and Honig's program for low-income fathers.

SEFAM originated at the University of Washington in Seattle and since 1985 has been located at the Merrywood School in Bellevue, Washington.[61] The program is based on three factors: support, education, and involvement. Support of the fathers is fostered through interaction with other fathers as they learn more about their own child. Convenient meeting times are arranged and codirected by a father and a special educator. These meetings are programmatic, extending fathers' knowledge in a selected area. A study assessing the direct and indirect effects of the program[62] found significant father outcomes of increased self-esteem and attributions of child competence and decreased stress and depression. Wives of program participants also benefited, with more positive feelings about themselves and their children. This program curriculum has been disseminated throughout the country through a videotape[63] as well as through written material[61] to further encourage paternal participation with special needs children.

The Bank Street College of Education established The Fatherhood Project[64] in 1981 to foster educational programming for males. The Project moved to the Families and Work Institute in 1989 and now conducts research on the conflict between the work and family responsibilities of men, presents seminars on the changing role of men in our society, and acts as a national clearinghouse for information related to fathers.

In order to facilitate fathers' therapeutic interaction with their special needs children, Revelj[65] conducted a direct hands-on program. She found that with initial flexibility in scheduling physical-therapy sessions with the father, she was able to gain program participation, which fathers interpreted as useful. Initial flexibility in scheduling appointments facilitated long-term involvement of fathers in the program. Techniques of direct modeling and written handouts reinforced the fathers' participation, helping them to modify their participation in exercise regimens and to continue these regimens at home. In a postprogram questionnaire, when asked which part of the program was the most beneficial, the fathers consistently said that the direct contact with the therapist was the most helpful, because it gave them an opportunity to clarify developmental questions and better understand the need for exercise.

A program developed and implemented by Honig and Pfannestiel[66] addressed the needs of low-income fathers and their infants. The program attempted to instruct the fathers in fetal and infant characteristics and behaviors and assist them in responding to child cues and states. Transportation was offered to fathers to facilitate their attendance at these instructional sessions. In addition, postpartum intervention was offered through neonatal assessment of the child. In a control group study, significantly improved quality of paternal interaction was found at 8 weeks with those fathers who had participated in the assessment of their child as a newborn.[67]

SUGGESTIONS

The concept of the "derelict dad" appears to be a myth. In reality, fathers who are available at all want to interact with their children. However, they may not know how, when, or where to be involved[68] or may not have been offered appropriate opportunities for involvement. To foster involvement, interventionists need to gain an appreciation of fathers as active participators in the care of their children. Fathers' interests need to be tapped, their energies channeled, and their skills refined. It is certain that their schedules need to be considered. Given this perspective, eight specific suggestions are presented for the interventionist to enhance the father's involvement and develop the father's commitment to the education of his child:

1. Recognize the unique role that the father has in the education of his special child. To provide fatherly advice and support, a male need not be the biologic father of a child. In the event that no father role exists for a particular child, the IFSP team may need to provide a male role model for the child. Although this is a controversial issue, the authors believe this course of action must be *at least considered* by the team for each child.
2. Determine the positive attributes, rather than problems, that the father assigns to his special child, and encourage a variety of normalizing activities to support and enhance those attributes. To establish the most effective communication, the case manager (service coordinator) may need to be selected by the family rather than appointed by the team.
3. Recognize cultural, traditional, and unique paternal perspectives and schedules that may lead to initial engagement and sustain long-term involvement with fathers. Evenings and Saturdays are the most amenable time for father support meetings, father-child play interactions, and therapist or teacher consultations with the father.
4. Accept male roles that may differ from your social and cultural perceptions of the father role. For example, fathers in a patriarchal culture are expected to manage the relationships of family members with the outside world. If questions are not directed initially to the father of such a family, future interaction with that family may be limited. Another example is the father who works all night and sleeps a good part of the day. Asking him to attend in IFSP conference held at noon will be inappropriate.
5. When possible, visit the family in the home and determine the unique interests, preferences, and roles of the father as they relate to the education of the child. The father may be handy as a carpenter, creating home conveniences and child equipment, yet never recognized by the team for his efforts.
6. Determine paternal perceptions as well as facts through the interview process. The decision-making IFSP process needs to incorporate the perceptions of the parents and eliminate the biases of the professionals.

7. Share relevant literature related to families with team members and administrators. When requested by families, provide concrete information on previous case results. Be specific in response to questions from the father.
8. Request administrators to use school facilities for extracurricular events such as father-child Saturday programs and evening group meetings, hire male personnel, provide transportation, and obtain support services such as recreational therapists to facilitate normalized learning opportunities for the child.

• • •

The myth of the "derelict dad" suggests that the extent of the father's role is to protect the mother while she cares for the child. Intervention teams have supported this myth by not establishing inclusion of the father in program planning as a priority. A review of the literature suggests that the reality is that fathers are an integral part of the family unit and as such are involved and want to share, if not assume, responsibility for their children. However, when the educational system mandates specific activities for fathers, it fails to recognize and use the unique knowledge, experience, and perspective of the father. Instead, the father may want to direct his own participation and at times even that of the team. It is the responsibility of therapists, teachers, and administrators alike to create environments that foster such meaningful paternal involvement in the development and education of children.

REFERENCES

1. Meyer DJ. Fathers of children with mental handicaps. In: Lamb ME, ed. *The Father's Role: Applied Perspectives.* New York, NY: John Wiley & Sons; 1986.
2. Education of the Handicapped Act Amendments of 1986 (PL 99-457). USC.
3. Bane MJ, Masnick G. *The Nations Families: 1960–1990.* Boston, Mass: Auburn House Publishers; 1980.
4. US Bureau of the Census. *Marital Status and Living Arrangements: March, 1984.* Current Population Reports, Series P-20, No 399. Washington, DC: Government Printing Office; 1985.
5. Adams PL, Milner JR, Schrepf NA. *Fatherless Children.* New York, NY: John Wiley & Sons; 1984.
6. Wylie P. *Generation of Vipers.* New York, NY: Farrar & Rinehart; 1942.
7. Bowlby J. *Maternal Care and Infant Health.* Geneva, Switzerland: World Health Organization; 1951.
8. Meerlo JAM. The psychological role of the father: The father cuts the cord. *Child Fam.* 1968; Spring: 102–116.
9. Crowe TK. Father involvement in early intervention programs. *Phys Ther Occup Ther Pediatr.* 1981;1:35–46.
10. Lamb ME, ed. *The Father's Role: Applied Perspectives.* New York, NY: John Wiley & Sons; 1986.

11. Ninio A, Rinott N. Fathers' involvement in the care of their infants and their attributions of cognitive competence to infants. *Child Dev.* 1988;59:652–663.
12. Bowen SM, Miller BC. Paternal attachment behavior as related to presence at delivery and preparenthood classes: A pilot study. *Nurs Res.* 1980;29:307–311.
13. Cranley MS. Roots of attachment: The relationship of parents with their unborn. *Birth Defects.* 1981;17:59–83.
14. Parke RD. *Fathers.* Cambridge, Mass: Harvard University Press; 1981.
15. Parke RD, Anderson ER. Fathers and their at-risk infants: Conceptual and empirical analyses. In: Berman PW, Pedersen FA, eds. *Men's Transitions to Parenthood: Longitudinal Studies of Early Family Experience.* Hillsdale, NJ: Erlbaum Associates; 1987.
16. Jones C. Father to infant attachment: Effects of early contact and characteristics of the infant. *Res Nurs Health.* 1981;4:193–200.
17. Parke RD, Sawin DB. The family in early infancy: Social interactional and attitudinal analyses. In: Pedersen FA, ed. *The Father-Infant Relationship: Observation Studies in a Family Context.* New York, NY: Praeger; 1980.
18. Harrison MJ. A comparison of parental interactions with term and preterm infants. *Res Nurs Health.* 1990;13:173–179.
19. Belsky J. The determinants of parenting: A process model. *Child Dev.* 1984;55:83–96.
20. Clarke-Stewart KA. And daddy makes three: The father's impact on mother and young child. *Child Dev.* 1978;49:466–479.
21. Field TM. Fathers' interactions with their high-risk infants. *Inf Mental Health J.* 1981;2:249–256.
22. Lamb ME, Frodi MA, Hwang C, Frodi M, Steinberg J. Mother- and father-infant interaction involving play and holding in traditional and nontraditional Swedish families. *Dev Psychol.* 1982;18:215–221.
23. Tomasello M, Conti-Ramsden G, Ewert B. Young children's conversations with their mothers and fathers: Differences in breakdown and repair. *J Child Lang.* 1990;17:115–130.
24. Ban PL, Lewis M. Mothers and fathers, girls and boys. Attachment behavior in the one-year-old. *Merrill-Palmer Q.* 1974;20:195–204.
25. Pleck JH. American fathering in historical perspective. In: Kimmel MS, ed. *Changing Men: New Directions in Research on Men and Masculinity.* Newbury, Calif: Sage; 1987.
26. MacNab RT. What do men want? Male rituals of initiation in group psychotherapy. *Int J Group Psychother.* 1990;40:139–154.
27. Hardin G. The tragedy of the commons. *Science.* 1968;162:1,243–1,248.
28. Mackey WC. *Fathering Behaviors: The Dynamics of the Man-Child Bond.* New York, NY: Plenum Press; 1985.
29. Pruett K. Oedipal configurations in young father-raised children. *Psychoanal Study Child.* 1985;40:435–456.
30. Breslau N, Salkever D, Staruch KS. Women's labor force activity and responsibilities for disabled dependents: A study of families with disabled children. *Health Soc Behav.* 1982;23:169–183.
31. Wikler L. Chronic stresses of families of mentally retarded children. *Family Relations.* 1981;30:281–288.
32. Garcia Coll GT. Developmental outcome of minority infants: A process-oriented look into our beginnings. *Child Dev.* 1990;61:270–289.
33. Bailey DB, Winton PJ, Rouse L, Turnbull AP. Family goals in infant intervention: Analysis and issues. *J Early Intervent.* 1990;14:15–26.

34. Sparling JW. The transdisciplinary approach with developmental disabilities. *Phys Ther Occup Ther Pediatr.* 1980;1:1–9.
35. Committee on Education and Labor. Education of the Handicapped Act Amendments of 1986: Report 99-860. Washington, DC: House of Representatives, September 22, 1986.
36. Bailey DB, Palsha SA, Huntington GS. Preservice preparation of special educators to serve infants with handicaps and their families: Current status and training needs. *J Early Intervent.* 1990;14:43–54.
37. Cochrane CG, Farley B, Wilhelm IJ. Preparation of physical therapists to work with handicapped infants and their families: Current status and training needs. *Phys Ther.* 1990;70:372–380.
38. Crais ER, Leonard CR. PL 99-457: Are speech-language pathologists prepared for the challenge? *J Am Speech Hear Assoc.* 1990;32:57–61.
39. Downey WS. PL 94-142 and PL 99-457: Challenges for pediatrics. *J Fla Med Assoc.* 1987;74:778–782.
40. Humphry R, Link S. Entry level preparation of occupational therapists to work in early intervention programs. *Am J Occup Ther.* 1990;44:828–833.
41. Deal AG, Dunst CJ, Trivette CM. A flexible and functional approach to developing individualized family support plans. *Inf Young Child.* 1989;1:32–43.
42. Johnson BH, McGonigel MJ, Kaufman RK, eds. *Guidelines and Recommended Practices for the Individualized Family Service Plan.* Chapel Hill, NC: National Early Childhood Technical Assistance System; 1989.
43. Gowen JW, Johnson-Martin N. Infant assessment and the individual family service plan. Paper presented at the 67th Annual Convention of the Council for Exceptional Children, San Francisco, California, April 3–7, 1989.
44. Linder TW. *Transdisciplinary Play-Based Assessment: A Functional Approach to Working with Young Children.* Baltimore, Md: Paul H. Brookes Publishing Co, 1990.
45. Winton PJ, Bailey DB. The family-focused interview: A collaborative mechanism for family assessment and goal setting. *J Div Early Child.* 1988;12:195–207.
46. Gonzalez S, Steinglass P, Reiss D. *Family-Centered Interventions for People with Chronic Disabilities: The Eight-Session Multiple Family Discussion Group Program.* Washington, DC: George Washington University Medical Center; 1987.
47. Rowan LE, Thorp EK, McCollum JA. An interdisciplinary practicum to foster infant-family and teaming competencies in speech-language pathologists. *Inf Young child.* 1990;3:58–66.
48. Cummings ST. The impact of the child's deficiency on the father: A study of fathers of mentally retarded and of chronically ill children. *Am J Orthopsych.* 1976;46:246–255.
49. Patterson JM, McCubbin HI, Warwick WJ. The impact of family functioning on health changes in children with cystic fibrosis. *Soc Sci Med.* 1990;31:159–164.
50. Ferrari M. Perceptions of social support by parents of chronically ill versus health children. *Child Health Care.* 1986;15:26–31.
51. Frey KS, Fewell RR, Vadasy PF. Parental adjustment and changes in child outcome among families of young handicapped children. *Top Early Child Spec Ed.* 1989;8:38–57.
52. Goldberg S, Morris P, Simmons RJ, Fowler RS, Levison H. Chronic illness in infancy and parenting stress: A comparison of three groups of parents. *J Pediatr Psychol.* 1990;15:347–358.
53. Damrosch SP, Perry LA. Self-reported adjustment, chronic sorrow, and coping of parents of children with Down syndrome. *Nurs Res.* 1989;38:25–30.

54. Levy-Shiff R, Hoffman MA, Mogilner S, Levinger S, Mogilner MB. Fathers' hospital visits to their preterm infants as a predictor of father-infant relationship and infant development. *Pediatrics.* 1990;86:289–293.

55. McCain GC. Family functioning 2 to 4 years after preterm birth. *J Pediatr Nurs.* 1990;5:97–104.

56. Ehrensaft M. Man, woman, and child: The shared parenting family. Paper presented at the Annual Convention of the Orthopsychiatric Association. New York, NY, April 20–24, 1985.

57. Lamb ME, Pleck JH, Levine JA. Effects of increased paternal involvement on fathers and mothers. In: Lewis C, O'Brien M, eds. *Reassessing Fatherhood: New Observations on Fathers and the Modern Family.* Beverly Hills, Calif: Sage; 1982.

58. Seymore C, Frothingham TE, MacMillan J, Durant RH. Child development knowledge, childrearing attitudes, and social support among first- and second-time adolescent mothers. *J Adolescent Health Care.* 1990;11:343–350.

59. Garcia Coll CT, Hoffman J, Oh W. The social ecology and early parenting of Caucasian adolescent mothers. *Child Dev.* 1987;58:955–963.

60. Unger DG, Wandersman, LP. The relation of family and partner support to the adjustment of adolescent mothers. *Child Dev.* 1990;59:1,056–1,060.

61. May J. *Fathers of Children with Special Needs: New Horizons.* Bethesda, Md: Association for the Care of Children's Health; 1990.

62. Vadasy PF, Fewell RR, Meyer DJ, et al. Supporting fathers of handicapped young children: Preliminary findings of program effects. *Anal Intervent Dev Disabil.* 1985;5:151–163.

63. SEFAM Family Support Program. *Special Kids, Special Dads—Fathers of Children with Disabilities.* Rockville, Md: Association for the Care of Children's Health; 1989.

64. Klinman D, Kohl R. *The Fatherhood Project: Fatherhood USA. The First National Guide to Programs, Services, and Resources for and about Fathers.* New York: Garland; 1984.

65. Revelj EO. Increasing fathers' participation in therapeutic intervention programs for exceptional children. Available on microfiche. ED 275110; Reston, Virginia; ERIC, 1985.

66. Honig AS, Pfannestiel A. Clinical issues in reaching low-income fathers with a program of "Information and Insights about Infants" (III). Paper presented at the Annual Meeting of the American Orthopsychiatric Association. San Francisco, California, March, 1988. Available on microfiche. ED 291474; Reston, Virginia: ERIC, 1988.

67. Beal JA. The effect on father-infant interaction of demonstrating the neonatal behavioral assessment scale. *Birth.* 1989;16:18–31.

68. Bristol M, Gallagher J. Research on fathers of young handicapped children. In: Gallagher J, Vietze P, eds. *Families of Handicapped Persons.* Baltimore, Md: Paul H Brookes; 1986.

The family-centered consultation model: Practical applications for professionals

Audrey Leviton, MSW
Program Manager, Child and Family Support Program

Mary Mueller, MSW
Senior Staff Coordinator, Child and Family Support Program

Cynthia Kauffman, MA
Director
Department for Family Support Services
Kennedy Institute
Baltimore, Maryland

IN THE PAST few years, professionals and parents of infants and toddlers with special needs have struggled to understand and put into practice the philosophy of family-centered care. Kennedy Institute's Department for Family Support Services defines family-centered care as a collaborative relationship between families and professionals in the continual pursuit of being responsive to the priorities and choices of families.[1] There has been considerable discussion of the major elements that comprise family-centered service provision. These include an emphasis on parental choice in the determination of services, the development of systems that are flexible and responsive to identified needs of the family, and comprehensive programs that address the needs of all family members.[2,3]

Recent national initiatives such as the Child and Adolescent Service System Program, Mental Health Initiative; and Public Law 101-239, the Title V, Maternal and Child Health Block Grant amendments are now requiring states to make family-centered care a reality. In particular, Part H of PL 99-457 necessitates the development of an Individualized Family Service Plan (IFSP) for families of infants and toddlers who are either developmentally disabled or at risk. The IFSP, a process for families and professionals to plan and organize services and resources, is based on the family-centered philosophy of parental choice and decision making.[4]

Converting traditional service systems to a model based on family-centered care will necessitate changes in the roles of professionals, as well as in the practices of agencies working with families. This article is designed to assist professionals and agency administrators who are interested in implementing family-centered care practices. A model for establishing parent-professional relationships and a number of practical suggestions for implementing family-centered services are provided.

HISTORY OF PARENT-PROFESSIONAL RELATIONSHIPS

Relationships between parents and professionals have undergone many transitions over the past century. In the early 1990s, professionals believed that parents

The authors wish to thank Michael Chapman, Larry Edelman, and Mary McGonigel for their comments and suggestions on previous drafts of this article.

Inf Young Children 1992; 4(3): 1–8

"weren't up to the task of raising disabled children,"[5(p77)] and encouraged the placement of children with disability in institutions. If parents decided to care for their child with special needs at home, they relied on informal support groups, because no formal public or private services were available. In the 1940s and 1950s, parents began to utilize these informal networks to organize large advocacy groups such as the National Association for Retarded Citizens and the United Cerebral Palsy Association.[6]

The efforts of parent advocacy organizations stimulated legislation such as the Education for All Handicapped Children Act of 1975 (PL 94-142) and the Education Amendments of 1986 (PL 99-457), which not only mandated services to children with special needs but also stressed the importance of a good parent-professional relationship. These legislative efforts required professionals to involve parents in the determination of services for their child with special needs.[7]

The shift toward increased parental involvement has generated renewed interest in defining different models for parent-professional relationships. Trivette, Deal, and Dunst have described a variety of possible professional roles, including advocate, counselor, catalyst, mediator, enabler, resource, consultant, and teacher.[8] Regardless of the specific role assumed by the professional, the literature frequently describes the parent-professional relationship as a collaborative and equal partnership in the identification and delivery of services.[9–11] Summers expanded this concept by stating that "families are not merely adjuncts or even partners in providing services for the child . . . families should be in charge of the whole process."[12(p9)]

THEORETICAL FRAMEWORK FOR PARENT-PROFESSIONAL RELATIONSHIPS

The Kennedy Institute's Department for Family Support Services in Baltimore, Maryland, has provided training, counseling, coordination, and financial support to families of children with special needs for more than 10 years. During this time, parents have assisted the Department in developing a model for parent-professional relationships. Parents have often expressed how much they value the professional's knowledge and clinical expertise in relation to their child with special needs. However, parents have also stated that only they have the necessary expertise to determine whether professional recommendations can be successfully incorporated into their own family's lifestyle.

As a result, parents and the staff of the Department for Family Support Services realized that the role of the professional should resemble that of a consultant to the parents. Operating as a consultant means that staff members recognize that "families are the real experts on their child and respect each family's values and preferences with regard to all decisions about services."[12(p9)] Dunst, Trivette, and Deal described the role of the consultant as providing parents with information that assists them in making informed decisions and enables them to utilize their natural networks (ie, friends, family, neighbors) more effectively.[13]

The Department for Family Support Services has chosen Blake and Mouton's "catalytic consultation model" as its framework for working with families.[14] A catalytic consultant acts as a change agent by increasing the pace and quality of changes that are already in process. The catalytic model was developed to assist businesses in situations in which power and authority were an issue.[14] In the business world, the catalytic consultant does not diagnose and recommend solutions, but rather assists clients in collecting pertinent information so that they may be more effective in their jobs.[14]

The Department for Family Support Services, in adapting this model of business consultation to human services professionals, assists parents in collecting information that supports them in making decisions that they feel are right for them. Implementing the catalytic model in human services necessitates a redefinition of the role of professionals working with families. Outlined in Table 1 is a comparison of the professional's role in traditional models of intervention with his or her role in the family-centered consultation model of intervention. Three stages of intervention are compared: determining the parent-professional relationship and goals, generating strategies to achieve goals, and decision making and service delivery.

Stage 1

In traditional models, the first stage of intervention begins with a professional assessment of the child's and the family's level of functioning. The relationship between parents and professionals is largely predetermined by the agency's service delivery model. For example, a parent may feel very overwhelmed and come to an agency requesting assistance. The agency, which provides clinical services, may offer counseling services to the family without exploring the need for concrete services such as respite care or day care.

In the family-centered consultation model, the parent-professional relationship is not predetermined. The parent chooses the role and the degree of involvement of professionals. The relationship begins with parents and professionals jointly providing information to assist the parents in making informed decisions about which services and resources they would like to receive. This process may or may not include an assessment of the child with special needs and the family. To assist parents in clarifying their goals, a number of family needs assessments have been developed.[2,15] Professionals may also use the following exploratory questions:

- In looking at all areas of your life, what would be most helpful to you as a way to reduce stress (eg, dinner out, camp for siblings, money)? What would strengthen the resources within your family?
- How would your family like our staff to be involved (eg, counseling, service coordination, advocacy, support, training, etc)?

Table 1. Comparison of a traditional service delivery model with the family-centered consultation model

Stages of intervention	*Traditional model*	*The family-centered consultation model*
1. Determining the parent–professional relationship and goals	The relationship between the parent and professional is predetermined by the agency's service delivery model.	The relationship between the parent and professional is not predetermined. The parent chooses the role and the degree of involvement of the professional.
	Typically, the relationship begins with an assessment of the child and family's level of functioning.	The relationship begins with parents and professionals jointly providing information to assist the parents in making informed decisions about which services and resources they would like to receive. This may or may not include an assessment of their child and family.
2. Generating strategies to achieve goals	Based on the assessment of the child and family's needs, the professional generates recommendations and strategies that he or she believes will be beneficial to the family.	Based on the family's interests and concerns, the professional meets with the family to jointly explore a variety of options for achieving goals. Although professionals discuss options, they avoid giving specific recommendations.
	These assessment findings and recommendations are then discussed with the parents.	These joint discussions result in having the parents formulate strategies to achieve goals that they feel will be most beneficial to their child and family.
3. Decision making and service delivery	Based on professionals' recommendations, parents either begin to receive services or must seek other alternatives.	Once parents have decided on a plan, they begin to receive services from professionals as requested.
	Throughout service delivery, the professional provides the agreed-on services. Because the flexibility of the professional's role tends to be limited by agency constraints, families may need to be referred elsewhere for related services.	Throughout the service delivery, the role of the professional may vary as the needs and interests of the child and family change. Families may request that professionals provide a range of services including training, therapy, advocacy, support, information, and coordination.

- What training and/or support can we provide to you as a parent that will help in meeting your child's and family's needs?

Some parents may have difficulty responding to these questions because their own needs (eg, shelter, food, drug rehabilitation, mental health counseling) are overwhelming. For these parents, it is necessary to explore options that may not necessitate their direct involvement. Parents under extreme stress may desire direct service options that do not require parental participation (eg, school, appropriate funding sources, respite care). Some of these parents may also choose to have extended family members or close friends participate in interventions for their child.

Stage 2

The second state in the parent-professional relationship is generating strategies to achieve goals. In the traditional model, professionals, based on their assessments, generate recommendations and strategies that they believe will be beneficial to the family. These assessment findings and recommendations are then discussed with the parents.

In the family-centered consultation model, the professional avoids giving specific recommendations. Instead, the professional provides information to address the parent's concerns and, on request, explores "all" possible options—not just the one that the professional believes would be most effective in achieving the family's goals. The professional must also examine options that are not available through his or her own program but may be obtained by referral to the community agencies. This exploration results in the parents formulating strategies to achieve goals that they feel will be most beneficial to their child and family.

To illustrate this, consider the role of a professional providing services to a family with a child with cerebral palsy who has extensive intervention needs. Although the most efficient way to provide this service may be through a school program, the parents are hesitant to send their child to school because of his or her young age. In the family-centered consultation model, the professional's role could be to assist the family by coordinating services that may provide less direct therapy to the child but are more in accordance with the family's life style and beliefs.

Stage 3

The final stage involves decision making and service delivery. Traditionally, the parent either accepts the recommended services or must seek other alternatives. If the parent and the professional agree to the plan, the professional provides the recommended services to achieve the jointly agreed-upon goals. Because the flexibility of the professional's role tends to be limited by agency constraints, families may need to be referred elsewhere for related services. For example, teachers, doctors, and therapists may not have the flexibility to provide advocacy and coordination.

In the family-centered consultation model, the parents and professionals continue exploring options until the family has designed a plan that meets their needs. Through service delivery, the role of the professional may vary as the needs and interests of the child and family change. Parents may request that professionals provide a range of services including training, therapy, advocacy, support, information, and coordination.[8]

PRACTICAL SUGGESTIONS FOR PUTTING FAMILY-CENTERED CARE INTO PRACTICE

Just as the role of the professional must change in a family-centered system, so must the guiding policies and operating practices of agencies working with families. Innovative policies and practices must be developed that support and enhance emerging changes in the relationship between parents and professionals. Agencies must examine the degree to which their programs adhere to family-centered principles such as parent-directed decision making; flexibility in time, place, and style of service delivery; and addressing the needs of all members, not just the child with special needs.[2,3]

The need for agencies to respond to families in such a flexible manner necessitates a similar flexibility and responsiveness to the needs of staff members providing services to these families (eg, flexible work schedules and openness to creative service delivery approaches). Agencies that are responsive to staff members and families often benefit by increased staff and consumer satisfaction and retention.

To illustrate how service providers can incorporate these principles of family-centered care, select examples are offered in four areas of service delivery: referral, assessments, paperwork, and meetings.

Referral

Beginning with the initial referral, opportunities should be provided for parental participation. The locus of control should remain with the parents. To accomplish this, agencies should

- provide parents with a simple referral process, with one telephone number where someone is always available to receive the referral;
- require only the amount of information necessary for services to be initiated; it should not be necessary for families to wait several months for services while records are being sent; and
- accept referrals either directly from parents or only from professionals who have already confirmed the parents' interest in being referred.

Assessment

When the parent has requested an assessment of his or her child's skills, this assessment should be completed in a family-centered manner. The team, consisting of the child's parents and the professionals conducting the assessment, must recognize the central role of the parent in the assessment process. This can be demonstrated in all three stages of the process: planning the assessment, conducting the assessment, and providing feedback.

Planning the assessment

In planning the assessment, agencies must develop policies and practices that enable parents to

- formulate their concerns and questions, with professional consultation;
- choose from a variety of assessment formats (ie, single discipline, arena, multidisciplinary, and interdisciplinary); if parents are interested in using a standardized assessment tool, a range of options should be discussed from which the parents can choose;
- choose the location (home, school, office) and time (day or evening) for the assessment based on their schedule and needs;
- plan the evaluation process with involved professionals (eg, what will occur; which friends, family members, and/or professionals they would like to attend; which toys should be utilized to best elicit their child's responses); and
- determine the role they will take in the assessment process, ranging from facilitator to observer; some parents may choose to conduct the assessment themselves with support and guidance from professionals, whereas others may be more comfortable with professional facilitation.

Conducting the assessment

In conducting the assessment, professionals should

- ask the parents, before starting the assessment, if there are any last-minute changes they would like to make in the assessment process;
- clearly identify all team members and their role in the assessment (through the use of name tags and/or a written list of participants);
- ask parents throughout the assessment if the evaluation is progressing in the way they had planned (eg, Is there anything we have left out? Is there a way to make your child more comfortable? Is there anything else you would like us to see?); and
- explain why specific skills are being elicited.

Providing feedback

In communicating with parents following the assessment, professionals should

- ask parents their reactions to the assessment (eg, What was your overall response to the assessment? Is this typical of your child? Were there mitigating factors that affected your child's performance?); the parents' responses should be incorporated into any written assessment;

- know that parental observations of their child's usual behaviors and skills often have greater validity than professionals' observations during the assessment; this should be reflected in the written assessment;
- inform parents of what is typically included in a written assessment and ask if there are additional areas that they would like addressed;
- provide feedback beginning with the family's stated priorities and focus on the strengths and concerns of the family throughout the feedback process;
- provide both verbal and written results to parents as soon as possible; oral feedback, provided immediately following the assessment, should be accompanied by an informal written summary for the parents' use at the time of the assessment;
- include practical suggestions in the assessment that would be helpful to parents and other involved professionals;
- refrain from the use of jargon in both verbal and written feedback;
- provide copies of assessments free of charge to parents; and
- schedule a follow-up telephone call or meeting with the parents to discuss any remaining questions; parents should feel free to invite anyone they feel should participate in this follow-up discussion.

Paperwork

In a family-centered system, paperwork should reflect the parents' pivotal role in all decision making. In order to do this, agencies should:

- identify the family, not just the child with a disability, as the consumer; a suggested method to accomplish this is labeling the records with the family's last name, the parent's name, or the "family of _____."
- ensure that all correspondence to referral sources, doctors, and other involved agencies is composed and sent jointly by the parents and agency; and
- ensure that all paperwork is free of jargon and completed in a timely fashion.

Meetings

Meetings between parents and professionals are an essential feature of a family-centered system. The degree to which a parent is an integral member of the team is often evidenced in how meetings are planned and conducted. It is helpful if one staff member is identified as the primary liaison for the parents.

Prior to the meeting

In planning the meeting, agencies must develop policies and practices that enable parents to

- determine the logistics, format, and agenda of the meeting (eg, location, time, participants, parental role); for example, parents may choose to chair the meeting at 7:00 PM in their own home in order to accommodate work and child-care needs; and

- obtain necessary information to assist in formulating questions and concerns that will be addressed at the meeting. Professionals can assist by ensuring that parents have copies of all reports, as well as a complete list of meeting participants (titles and telephone numbers).

During the meeting

During the meeting, professionals should

- create a comfortable atmosphere in which parents are not treated differently from other team members; all team members, including the parents, should gather in the same room on arrival, and team members should wear name tags and should address one another with the same level of formality (ie, Mr or Mrs, or first names); Professionals should not address or refer to parents as "Mom" or "Dad," which immediately defines the relationships as unequal;
- begin the meeting by having either the parents or their liaison state the family's goals for the meeting;
- build on the strengths of the entire team (eg, family, professionals, child) to develop a plan that maximizes the potential of all participants;
- provide opportunities, if requested by the parents, to discuss and address concerns relating to other family members, not solely the child with special needs;
- review the initially stated family goals to see that they have been addressed to the parent's satisfaction; and
- ensure continued team commitment to agreed-upon goals by distributing minutes to all team members, including the parents. Professionals should acknowledge the continued availability of all other team members to the family.

• • •

Parents and professionals may be working together on the same issue but often from very different perspectives. The words of Peter Cumming, a parent writing about his dying son, powerfully illuminate the differing viewpoints of parents and professionals:

> This is our child. This is your patient.
> This is our life. This is your work.
> This is the creation of our love. This is a problem for you to solve.
> This is our only Paul. This is one of your many patients.[16(p30)]

Although differing perspectives can sometimes present obstacles in working together as a team, they can also provide opportunities for both professionals and parents to learn from one another. Parents value the knowledge and clinical expertise of involved professionals. Professionals must also learn to value the parent's expertise in knowing what is best for their child and family.

The family-centered consultation model recognizes that the parent's expertise, not the professional's, is the foundation for decision making. The challenge for professionals is to learn how to utilize their expertise within this framework of parent-directed decision making. The family-centered consultation model and the practical suggestions provided in this article offer one way to meet this challenge.

REFERENCES

1. Edelman L. *Recognizing Family-Centered Care: A Group Exercise-Facilitator's Guide.* Baltimore, Md: Project Copernicus, The Kennedy Institute; 1991.
2. Shelton T, Jeppson E, Johnson B. *Family-Centered Care for Children with Special Health Care Needs.* Bethesda, Md: National Center for Family-Centered Care, Association for the Care of Children's Health; 1989.
3. Frieser B, Griesbach J, Jacobs J, Katz-Leavy J, Olson D. Improving services for families. *Children Today.* 1988;17(4):18–22.
4. Johnson B, McGonigel M, Kaufmann R. *Guidelines and Recommended Practices for the Individualized Family Service Plan.* Washington, DC: Association for the Care of Children's Health and National Early Childhood Technical Assistance System; 1989.
5. Springen K, Kantrowitz B. The long goodbye. *Newsweek,* 27 October 1990;77–80.
6. Kirk S, Gallagher J. *Educating Exceptional Children.* Boston, Mass: Houghton Mifflin; 1986.
7. Burnim I. *Strengthening the Role of Families in State's Early Intervention Systems.* Washington, DC: Mental Health Law Project; 1990.
8. Trivette C, Deal A, Dunst C. Family needs, sources of support, and professional roles: Critical elements of family systems assessment and intervention. *Diagnostique.* 1986;11(3–4):246–267.
9. Brewer E, McPherson M, Magrab P, Hutchins V. Family centered, community-based coordinated care for children with special health care needs. *Pediatrics.* 1989;83(6):1,055–1,060.
10. Gittler J. *Community-Based Service Systems for Children with Special Health Needs and Their Families.* Iowa City, Iowa: University of Iowa, National Maternal and Child Health Resource Center; 1988.
11. Bazyk S. Changes in attitudes and beliefs regarding parent participation and home programs: An update. *Am J Occup Ther.* 1989;443(11):723–728.
12. Summers JA. Family-centered intervention: Issues and opportunities. In: *Families and Early Intervention, Impact.* Minneapolis, Minnesota: University of Minnesota Institute on Community Integration; 1989.
13. Dunst CJ, Trivette CM, Deal AG. *Enabling and Empowering Families.* Cambridge, Mass: Brookline Books; 1988.
14. Blake R, Mouton J. *Consultation: A Handbook for Individual and Organizational Development.* 2nd ed. Reading, Mass: Addison-Wesley; 1983.
15. Bailey D, Simeonnson R. *The Family Needs Survey.* Chapel Hill, NC: University of North Carolina, Frank Porter Graham Child Development Center, CIREEH.
16. Cumming P. This is our child, this is your patient. *Caring Mag.* 1986;6(11):30.

Family–provider relationships: The basis of all interventions

Barbara Kalmanson, PhD
Staff Psychologist

Stephen Seligman, DMH
Associate Clinical Professor
Infant–Parent Program
Department of Psychiatry
San Francisco General Hospital
University of California, San Francisco
San Francisco, California

IN THE LAST two decades, professionals working with infants and young children have come to see them in a new way. The world of the infant is now seen as one of great complexity, organization, and, most important, human relatedness. This new look is reshaping such fields as infant development, early education, developmental pediatrics, infant mental health, and many others. This article elaborates some of the most important implications for assessment and intervention that have emerged from this new approach. Our overarching emphasis is the importance of relationships, both infant–parent relationships and provider–family relationships, in determining the nature and outcome of development in general and interventions in particular. We begin by briefly outlining some of the most essential findings of recent infant observation research. We then present a framework for conceptualizing the working relationship between service providers and families, and we conclude by describing techniques for building working alliances with families. Strong working alliances are essential for providers in gathering information and planning and implementing interventions.

RECENT INFANT OBSERVATION RESEARCH: THE EMERGENCE OF A RELATIONSHIP-BASED APPROACH

The recent explosion of developmental research about infant development has shed light on the importance of early experience for all children. Although their obvious vulnerability and dependence has not been dismissed, infants' inborn social and emotional abilities have led to an emphasis on relationship-based interventions.[1–3]

Early research established that infants are born with preprogrammed abilities to signal and respond to social stimuli. For example, newborns prefer human faces to other sights and high-pitched human voices to other sounds, and often they can recognize their mothers' voices immediately after birth. These abilities mature rapidly in the context of caregiving relationships, giving the process of infant development its unique emotional appeal, whether in the newborn nursery, classroom, medical examining room, or even the supermarket. Essential aspects of early relatedness, such as bonding[4] and attachment,[5] have now been described in compelling and clinically useful ways.

Currently, these findings and others have converged in a general consensus among infant clinician-researchers that relationships are the organizing focus of

Inf Young Children 1992; 4(4): 46–52

all early development.[3,6–8] Emotional relatedness, for example, is a requirement for healthy physical development, as evidenced in the common causes of nonorganic failure to thrive.[9,10] Infants are dependent on their environment for love and care as well as physical support; these needs cannot be separated. Similarly, cognitive development and relationships are intertwined. Early caregiving relationships and, later, relationships with peers and teachers are the context within which growth takes place. Without the essential confidence that comes from the earliest experiences of other people's responsiveness, children do not feel the senses of vitality, effectiveness, and self-esteem that underlie exploration and both intellectual and motor development.

From the beginning, then, infants and parents are involved in dynamic, interactive relationship systems that integrate all spheres of development. Within these systems, both infants and parents play their unique roles, and different abilities and capacities may be considered separately. All diagnosis and intervention, however, whether educational, medical, social, or psychologic, must take the caregiving relationship into account. In addition, family structure and socioeconomic and cultural issues must not be overlooked.

Relationships and individual differences: Temperament and other constitutional variables

Within the relationship context, all infants are involved in ongoing processes of evoking and responding to care. However, infants show substantial individual differences from birth. They are born with unique temperamental characteristics, behavioral traits, and styles of responding to stimuli. Several dimensions of such differences have been described, including activity level, sensory threshold and responsiveness, curiosity, irritability, soothability, and the capacity to signal one's own needs and inner states.[7,11,12]

The importance of the infant–parent match

These differences have fundamental effects on caregiving relationships. Each infant has a particular style of interacting with the environment; each parent must adapt to the infant's individuality, and vice versa. Subtle variations in the infant's signaling style (eg, intensity and duration of crying and facial expression) and sensitivity to stimuli, for example, can create problems for some parent–infant pairs.

Parents also bring their own personal styles and personalities to the parenting situation, including such factors as their own experiences as children, capacity for empathic response, self-esteem, and socioeconomic and cultural dynamics. With an infant who is difficult to comfort, for example, a fragile, inexperienced mother who is sensitive to rejection or uncertain of her capacities to provide adequate care may withdraw in anger, frustration, or depression, whereas a more experienced parent with a reservoir of parenting success and self-esteem might patiently wait for the infant to become calm while taking subtle steps to enhance the infant's sense of organization and protection. With the withdrawing parent, a mutually reinforcing system of ineffectuality could develop, which could have profoundly negative consequences for both infant and parent.

Ultimately, the fit between the infant and the caregivers is more important than the attributes of either of them. This perspective, that no single factor in the evolving developmental system can be considered without reference to the other factors with which it is interacting, has been called the transactional approach.[13]

Intervention and the infant–parent match

Whether a particular intervention is focused on the infant, parent, or both, it will have effects on all aspects of the infant's and family's lives. Professionals should take a comprehensive and thoughtful approach that takes the complex impact of their interventions on developmental systems into account. Interdisciplinary collaboration is often exceptionally useful.

At the same time, however, it will be essential to acknowledge our own limitations. Many of the effects of interventions cannot be predicted, and most current intervention contexts are administratively and financially constrained. When such limitations are not discussed, both among colleagues and between providers and clients, unstated frustrations may impede both working relationships and technical interventions.

THE IMPORTANCE OF WORKING RELATIONSHIPS: IMPLICATIONS FOR DIAGNOSIS AND INTERVENTION

Providers must pay careful attention to their own relationships with the infants and families with whom they are working. Without a minimal working alliance with the families, interventions, in whatever field, cannot be successful. This will be true for even the most simple interventions. The prescription of an antibiotic for an infant with an infection, for example, will not work unless the parents have enough confidence in their pediatric providers to administer the medication. They must also have the psychosocial skills to comply with dosage schedules and the like, and the economic system must be able to make the medication available to them. Fortunately, we are often able to take such factors for granted, but in all fields even the most specific technical interventions will be enhanced when providers are sensitive to both infant–parent and parent–provider relationships.[14] Such considerations have recently received more attention in such fields as special education and pediatrics, and new legislation has shown increasing sensitivity in this area.

The success of all interventions will rest on the quality of provider–family relationships, even when the relationship itself is not the focus of the intervention. Effective and sympathetic working relationships enhance parents' all too often neglected recognition that it is their efforts that are ultimately most important to their infants. Families with special needs often feel that their particular difficulties set them apart from others, and a good relationship with a professional can enhance the sense of being understood and supported. This, in turn, can lead to changes in the parent–child relationship.[15,16]

Because parents' relationships with providers often parallel their relationships with their children, we can learn important lessons about parents' and infants' experiences of one another by observing the issues that arise in the provider–family arena. Sometimes, these issues will also reflect the parents' childhood experiences with their own parents. In a surprising number of cases, parents treat their infants as their parents treated them, and they expect professionals to act in a similar way. The offer of a different kind of relationship that accompanies sensitively presented interventions can spark changes in parents' characteristic modes of relationship. These changes can have enduring effects, especially when they are amplified by correlated changes in the infant–parent relationship. In some cases, the evocation of the parental "ghosts in the nursery" can be so dramatic that more intensive psychotherapeutic techniques must be used, but in many situations a nonpsychotherapeutic intervention can have a significant impact on the caregiving relationship.[1,17] Although such issues must be handled with exceptional tact and sensitivity, being involved in such emotional transformations can be especially gratifying for providers.

SPECIFIC TECHNIQUES FOR BUILDING A WORKING RELATIONSHIP

Observing and following the child's lead

Direct observation of an infant or young child is often the best place to start building a productive and trusting relationship with a family. It is widely acknowledged that observation provides opportunities to assess family interaction, parent–child relationships, and the child's capacities. Observation, however, also enables providers to convey a sense of appreciation of both parents' and children's experiences. Careful attention to the child's activities yields knowledge of the child's ways of eliciting interaction and responding to family members at the same time that it creates opportunities for discussing this knowledge with them. Parents will feel concretely understood when they sense the providers' empathy for both their own and their children's inner experience of everyday events as they unfold. This creates possibilities for emotional reflection and potential for psychologic change.

In addition, emphasizing observation will set a tone for future work with the family. If we watch and listen, the child will tell us what he or she needs. Our confidence in this approach helps parents begin to learn from their children.

Home visiting

Visiting the family at home and following the child's daily activities is the most informative method of gathering information. A number of questions can be answered that would otherwise remain obscure: Who attends to this child, and under what circumstances? How much freedom and restriction does the child experience? To what level of stimulation is the child exposed? Home visits have the benefit of letting us see the child without the distortions imposed by the unfamiliarity of new people and places.

Offering to come to the family home often convinces the family of the provider's willingness to anticipate its needs because the practitioner is showing in action that he or she understands how difficult it may be for a family that is already stressed to make the arrangements necessary to avail itself of services. Even when home visits are not possible, for example because of agency constraints or a family's sensitivity about housing conditions, naturalistic observation should not be abandoned. A playroom can be set up for families to meet comfortably in a homelike environment, where the advantages of observing by following the child's lead can still be gained. Although more formal assessment techniques and history taking are often useful, observation should always be given a high priority.

Obtaining developmental history

Observation gives us a different kind of information than traditional history taking and formal testing. Information obtained from history taken in a checklist format often feels sketchy and distant and can be tainted by parents' distortions and lapses in memory.[1,18] Historical and developmental information obtained in the context of observing the child in interaction yields a more accurate representation of the past and of the relationship of the past to the present. Recurring feelings associated with the earlier experiences create rich opportunities for discussion and furnish the provider with the emotional underpinnings of developmental data.

Direct observation differs from formal testing because one is able to assess a child's development in the context of the relationships in which the child's capacities have unfolded thus far. Observing how a child's way of learning about and having an effect on the world is facilitated or impeded by parents' caregiving approaches puts a provider in a better position to know the strengths and vulnerabilities of the caregivers in relation to the child's current development. Such observations are often immediately useful in understanding parents' frustration around particular developmental challenges or caregiving routines and in creating fertile ground for developmental guidance and intervention planning.

The meaning of the child's behavior

When providers follow the child's lead while observing, parents learn that the child's behavior is important. Parents can be helped to understand that the child's behavior has meaning that can be interpreted and understood in collaborative efforts to assist development.When parents think of intervenors as doing things to the child rather than understanding what the child is doing, they will model their interactions with the child on this more intrusive style of interaction, even when it feels foreign to them. By watching and exploring the meaning of the child's behavior, a provider can formulate a treatment plan with parents that is respectful of the child's rhythms and idiosyncracies as well as of the parents' caregiving style. When parents who have been intrusive or insensitive learn to take the lead from the child, they have new tools for understanding the child's sometimes incomprehensible behavior and figuring out their own intervention strategies. Ideally, providers will follow the lead of both parents and children and will work to set up an atmosphere of empathy and trust that will foster support and progressive change.

Eliciting parents' perceptions of their child

The subjective experience of parents and infants, rather than their objective behavior, should be the focus of the intervention. By eliciting parents' perceptions of what their child is doing and why the child is behaving in a particular way, a provider can gain essential information about how the parents understand the child's behavior. Earning parents' trust and belief that a provider can genuinely understand them in relation to their child is an essential element in establishing a working alliance.

Often, parents interpret the child's behavior in a variety of ways that reflect their personal conflicts. At times, parents may take a child's difficulties as evidence of personal shortcomings. In addition, problematic qualities in the parents' own personalities may be attributed to the child, as when a child is thought to be provocative or is caricatured as defective. Providers can free parents to reconsider such misperceptions about the child only by first understanding how they came to their point of view and how these misperceptions have affected the infant–parent relationship. By eliciting parents' perceptions and empathizing with their experience of the child, the provider frees the parent to empathize with their child's experience, and rather than personalize the meaning of the child's behavior, the parents are able to ally themselves with the provider in their work together on the child's behalf.

For example, the parents of a learning-disabled preschooler perceived their child as lazy, despite the fact that he was quite active at times, because they had to force him to do certain things. Only after lengthy discussion of their own feelings about pushing him, their impatience with his testing them, and the kinds of things he was and was not lazy about were the parents able to recognize particular patterns and think that their son's laziness reflected a constitutional sensitivity in a particular sensory pathway.

Requesting and giving information

Providers should always be extremely sensitive to parents' intense emotions about their children, especially in the unusually stressful situations accompanying the idiosyncratic development of children with special needs. In such circumstances, meeting with a provider creates anxiety, even when the practitioner's intentions and skills are of the highest quality.

Often, parents are confused or intimidated by professional jargon, and their feelings about participating in a working relationship are affected. Signs of this phenomenon are often overlooked; these include parents' becoming quiet during sessions, avoiding obvious questions, or failing to follow through with recommendations to which they have appeared to agree.

Providers should always describe behavior and recommendations in clear and simple terms and then invite parents to ask questions and to ask for clarification. If professionals anticipate with parents that what they say may not always be clear, parents will feel more able to ask questions and express their feelings.

As one talks with parents, then, it is helpful to create a shared language for discussing feelings and the meanings of the child's behavior. Shared language can be developed by carefully clarifying and defining the behaviors and activities one sees and parents report, including tactfully calling attention to discrepancies. For example, when a parent reports that his daughter was toilet trained at 2, the parent and provider may each have a different image. By exploring specific details of the father's account of how training took place, a provider can gather vital information that would not otherwise come to light.

Intrusiveness versus gathering information

Sometimes providers worry that they will be seen as intruding on or criticizing the family if they ask questions. However, questions can be used nonjudgmentally and with a genuine interest in whatever response is forthcoming. In one situation, for example, a young mother confessed that she used a belt to discipline her toddler and commented, "They call it child abuse." Concerned about being seen as punitive, the provider asked no further questions, and an uneasy silence waited to be broken by the toddler's play. Alternatively, sympathetic curiosity about who is calling it abuse and how the mother feels about the belt and the accusation could have brought the parent and practitioner closer together.

The provider's support and empathy for each family member help parents trust that their subjective experience is being understood. Support can take many forms, from confirming a parent's feelings and perceptions to providing concrete support around particular tasks related to the child's care. For some parents, concrete support is the only way to provide an experience of relationships as helpful rather than disappointing.

Developmental guidance

Despite our understanding of what we observe, parents often remain mystified by their children. This is especially true in the face of the idiosyncratic patterns of development in the vulnerable child. Parents often need help sorting out what expectations are realistic for their child and in placing specific behaviors in a developmental context.

The particular style with which this kind of information is given can determine the parent's experience of such offers of help. Surprisingly, directive, didactic approaches often fall on deaf ears. Parents receiving services regarding their child's development or their child-rearing approach are already sensitive about providing effective parenting and so are particularly likely to feel criticized. Tact is therefore especially important in these situations. Optimally, developmental guidance should acknowledge how puzzling a child's behavior can be, find kernels of important data in parents' reports, and confirm them as experts about their own children.

Pitfalls for providers

In their attempts to offer technical assistance, providers sometimes overlook the idiosyncratic personalities and needs of both parents and infants and instead attempt to impose their own way of thinking about the infant's difficulties on the family. As individuals and in their relationships, parents and infants present their own unique styles of coping with the challenges of ordinary development as well as with the extraordinary demands presented by children's special physical and developmental concerns. Professionals should always monitor both parents' and infants' reactions to their interventions and allow subsequent interventions to be guided by the responses offered. Because such cues are sometimes subtle, providers should always be as sensitive as possible to the ongoing feel of the evolving intervention relationship.

Tracking the emotional nuances of the working relationship while pursuing particular technical goals is a challenging task for professionals. This task is further complicated by the fact that providers' own emotional reactions can sometimes impede their sensitivity to the families whom they are trying to help. For example, professionals' most earnest wishes to help infants and their families can turn to frustration when their treatment goals are not met as rapidly as they might expect; such frustration can contribute to a sense of resentment and mutual disappointment that will impede the emergence of whatever potentials for progress remain.

In addition, the specific relationship issues that families bring to the intervention situation evoke negative feelings that are linked to providers' own personal issues and conflicts. Working with infants and their families, especially where children have special needs, can be emotionally provocative and challenge longstanding defenses and coping strategies for professionals as well as for parents. Ideally, such reactions should be treated as data for enhancing the intervention relationship and should be carefully considered. Tolerating and examining these feelings will generally prove more useful than succumbing to the temptations to suppress and censor them or to act quickly upon them.

REFERENCES

1. Fraiberg S. *Clinical Studies in Infant Mental Health: The First Year of Life.* New York, NY: Basic Books; 1980.
2. Lieberman AF, Pawl JH. Infant-parent psychotherapy. In: Zeanah C, Toth S, eds. *Handbook of Infant Mental Health.* New York, NY: Guilford. In press.
3. Sameroff AJ, Emde RN. *Relationship Disturbances in Early Childhood: A Developmental Approach.* New York, NY: Basic Books; 1989.
4. Klaus MH, Jerauld R, Kreger N, McAltine W, Steffa M, Kennell JH. Maternal attachment: Importance of the first post-partum days. *N Engl J Med.* 1972;286:460–463.
5. Bowlby J. *Attachment and Loss.* New York, NY: Basic Books; 1969;1.
6. Brazelton TB, Cramer BG. *The Earliest Relationship: Parents, Infants and the Drama of Early Attachment.* Reading, Mass: Addison-Wesley; 1990.
7. Greenspan S. *Psychopathology and Adaptation in Infancy and Early Childhood: Principles of Clinical Diagnosis and Preventive Intervention.* New York, NY: International Universities Press; 1981.
8. Stern DN. *The Interpersonal World of the Infant.* New York, NY: Basic Books; 1985.
9. Drotar D, Malone C, Negray J. Environmentally based failure to thrive and children's intellectual developmental. *J Clin Child Psychol.* 1980;9:236–240.
10. Lieberman AF, Birch M. The etiology of failure to thrive: An interactional developmental approach. In: Drotar D, ed. *New Directions in Failure to Thrive: Research and Clinical Practice.* New York, NY: Plenum; 1985.
11. Korner AF. Individual differences at birth: Implications for early experience and later development. *Am J Orthopsychiatr.* 1971;41:608–619.
12. Thomas A, Chess S, Birch HG. *Temperament and Behavior Disorders in Children.* New York, NY: New York University Press; 1968.

13. Sameroff AJ, Chandler MJ. Reproductive risk and the continuum of caretaking casualty. In: Horowitz FD, ed. *Review of Child Development Research.* Chicago, Ill: University Press; 1975;4.

14. Seligman S, Pawl J. Impediments to the formation of the working alliance in infant-parent psychotherapy. In: Call JH, Galenson E, Tyson RL, eds. *Frontiers of Infant Psychiatry.* New York, NY: Basic Books; 1984;2.

15. Seligman S. The effect of intervention relationships on parent-infant relationships: Perspectives from infant observation research and psychoanalysis. Presented at the Reginald S, Lourie Scientific Forum; May 1989; Washington, DC.

16. Heinicke CI, Beckwith L, Thompson A. Early intervention in the family system: A framework and a review. *Infant Ment Health J.* 1988;9:111–141.

17. Fraiberg S, Adelson E, Shapiro V. Ghosts in the nursery: A psychoanalytic approach to the problem of impaired infant-mother relationships. *J Am Acad Child Psychiatr.* 1975;14:387–422.

18. McCune L, Kalmanson B, Fleck MB, Glazewski B, Sillari J. An interdisciplinary model of infant assessment. In Meisels SJ, Shonkoff JP, eds. *Handbook of Early Intervention.* New York, NY: Cambridge University Press; 1990.

Building family-centered practices in early intervention: A team-based model for change

Donald B. Bailey, Jr, PhD
Director

P.J. McWilliam, PhD
Research Associate

Pamela J. Winton, PhD
Research Investigator
Frank Porter Graham Child Development Center
University of North Carolina at Chapel Hill
Chapel Hill, North Carolina

EARLY INTERVENTION programs serving infants and toddlers with disabilities face significant challenges in implementing family-centered services. First, it appears that most programs currently are offering services that are primarily child focused rather than family centered. For example, three studies[1–3] surveying early intervention professionals in 10 states have documented that professionals perceive a substantial discrepancy between typical and ideal practices in working with families due primarily to lack of administrative support, limited time and resources, and perceived lack of interest or skills on the part of families. Similar studies[4,5] in hospital settings have indicated that the ideals of family-centered care are sometimes discrepant with perceived roles of medical personnel.

A second barrier to family-centered services is lack of appropriate training. Most early intervention professionals have received little training in working with families[6] and perceive their skills to be stronger in working with children.[7] Although early intervention professionals appear to value work roles related to family support, they have a number of concerns about how a family-centered philosophy would be operationalized and how it would affect themselves, the teams(s) on which they work, and the families and children they serve.[7]

A third part of the challenge of implementing family-centered approaches stems from lack of a clear definition of family-centered care. Although helpful definitions have been offered,[8] it has become clear that family-centered care is a concept based on basic values and philosophic assumptions (eg, family support, families as decision makers, empowerment, coordinated services, normalization, cultural sensitivity), rather than a fixed set of services or a step-by-step procedure. Even the federal regulations accompanying Public Law 99-457 reflect the relative nature of the concept, providing considerable freedom for communities and states to establish parameters and procedures for family-centered services.

These factors (lack of training, child-focused practices, professional attitudes, administrative barriers, lack of a clearly articulated set of procedures) represent a

---

Preparation of this article was supported in part by grant no. G0087C3064, Special Education Program, Office of Special Education and Rehabilitative Services, US Department of Education.

Inf Young Children 1992; 5(1): 73–82

formidable challenge to practitioners, administrators, and trainers. Meaningful reform of early intervention practices will be unlikely if change facilitators attempt to rely on traditional strategies such as coursework, workshops, or changes in rules and regulations. Real change will occur only when a comprehensive, long-term, systematic approach is taken and when those who will be affected by change participate in decisions about its implementation.[9]

Drawing on this background, the authors have developed a decision-making model that provides early intervention teams a structure and framework for becoming more family centered in their work.[10] This article outlines the components of the model and presents the rationale for each component.

ASSUMPTIONS UNDERLYING THE MODEL

The model is based on several assumptions about the change process drawn from literature on organizational change and school reform[10–13]:

- Change is always a difficult process; it is especially challenging when the change involves an orientation that differs substantially from current practices.
- Change is a gradual, long-term process that will require ongoing staff development activities that become institutionalized as a regular part of the program planning process.
- Change is more likely to occur if small, easy to accomplish objectives are identified that allow personnel to blend new ideas with existing practices.
- When professionals work together as teams, training and decision making must occur at the team level so that all team members develop a shared perspective on change.
- A major goal of training should be to empower team members so that they can assess needs for change and identify strategies for enhancing it.
- When possible and appropriate, consumers of services should be given opportunities to provide input to decisions about changes to be made.

Based on these assumptions, a workshop format was developed as the initial step in implementing a family-centered approach in early intervention. Although workshops alone are not likely to result in radical changes in the way professionals work with families, they do provide a format in which significant planning can occur. The goal of the workshop, which typically lasts 4 days, is to provide the necessary information and a structure in which local early intervention teams jointly describe current practices, identify desired changes, and establish goals. The outcome of the workshop is a specific plan describing goals, resources, and strategies for implementing family-centered practices. To be successful, the workshop must be followed by an extended period of time in which teams engage in a variety of activities designed to achieve the goals identified. The five components of the workshop described in this article are (1) team-based training, (2) parent participation, (3) a decision-oriented format, (4) guided decision-making and goal-setting activities, and (5) effective leadership.

TEAM-BASED TRAINING

Many current efforts at school reform rely on school-based[14] or site-based[15] management strategies. Inherent in these approaches are two key principles: local autonomy and shared decision making.[14] Local autonomy assumes that communities vary in needs and resources, and thus they should be allowed to make decisions, and allocate services in ways that best reflect community priorities, subject of course to state or federal regulations and standards for quality. Shared decision making assumes that practicing professionals should have a voice in decisions about program practices. When professionals who are responsible for providing services are allowed to participate in significant decisions about intervention practices, they develop "ownership" of the change and are more likely to implement new practices.[11] For example, a recent study[16] demonstrated that a model of inservice training in which teachers generated their own ideas for change was effective in helping them embed instruction related to Individual Education Programs (IEPs) into regular classroom routines.

Two fundamental assumptions about early intervention programs and a family-centered approach are central to this model of training. First, providing support to families should be part of each professional's work. This assumption means that each professional will need to examine current roles and relationships with families and identify practices that may need to change in order to be more responsive to family needs and priorities. The second assumption is that moving to family-centered services must also be a decision that is made by the team as a whole. Without a shared commitment to families, services are likely to be fragmented and inconsistent. Families will get one message from some team members and another message from others. Part of being family centered is the provision of coordinated services based on a shared philosophy of how families are involved in every aspect of service delivery, whether it be assessment, child care, family support, therapeutic services, case management, team meetings, or consultation.

Some workshops are directed toward specific individuals for the purpose of teaching specific skills. Such an approach will not work, however, if the training involves issues that affect all team members in some way. The activities in this workshop assume that all team members are present during the entire set of activities. It is also assumed that key administrators are there. Research[1–5] has clearly documented that professionals who actually provide services to children and families perceive substantial administrative barriers to implementing a family-centered approach. By participating jointly in the workshop, administrators send a message to service providers that they endorse the decision-making activities being conducted and that they are willing to work with professionals to change program practices. Such participation is essential, because teams, as a result of the workshop, will often make decisions that will require administrative support. Also, by being present during the activities, administrators will gain a better understanding of the rationale behind the decisions made and can be a part of the decision-making process.

FAMILY PARTICIPATION

A second component of the model is family participation in all workshop activities. Several benefits of involving consumers in decisions about program policies have been suggested.[17,18] Because families are the primary recipients of a family-centered approach to services, it seems only logical that they should have input into how those services are to be provided. Including families in the activities should increase the likelihood that the decisions are acceptable to families. Family members can present a perspective that professionals cannot. Furthermore, including families in workshop activities is consistent with a family-centered philosophy and establishes a precedent for families serving in a role of decision maker.

In order to assess the effects and perceptions of parent participation in these activities, a study[19] was conducted in which two sets of workshops were held, one in which parents were invited to attend along with professionals and one that was attended only by professionals. The results indicated that parents influenced the extent to which professionals perceived a need for change in program practices. Professionals participating in a workshop where parents attended identified more areas of practice in which change was needed than professionals attending a workshop without parents present. Parents and professionals in the workshop where parents attended were positive about the experience; professionals who attended the workshop without parents felt strongly that parents should have been there.

A DECISION-ORIENTED FORMAT

The primary functions of the workshop are self-examination, decision making, and goal setting; the ultimate goal is for each team to create a unique plan for change. The role of the trainer or facilitator is to provide a framework and a context in which professionals examine program practices as they relate to a family-centered approach. Through this process of self-examination, professionals describe what their program is doing right now, how that compares to a family-centered approach, and whether a change is needed. Six key questions are addressed (see the Appendix):

1. What is our philosophy about working with families?
2. How will we involve families in child assessment?
3. How will we assess family needs and resources?
4. How will we involve families in team meetings and decision making?
5. How will we write family goals and the Individualized Family Service Plan (IFSP)? and
6. How will we implement the IFSP and provide case management?

The activities of the workshop are designed around these key questions, with approximately a half day devoted to each question. In addition, within each key question are embedded a series of challenge questions regarding various program practices and procedures (Appendix). The purpose of the challenge questions is to provide specific examples of issues that could be considered within each broad area.

A central aspect of the decision-making process is goal setting. Ample research in business and education suggests that when organizations set specific goals, change is more likely to occur. Because of the sometimes nebulous nature of a family-centered approach to services, the setting of specific goals becomes even more important. Thus the primary outcome of the workshop activities is an identification of needed areas of change and a ranking of priorities related to each key question.

GUIDED DECISION-MAKING ACTIVITIES

Making informed decisions about program change requires information about best practices, rules and regulations that need to be followed, and a structure for guiding group discussion and decision-making activities. In order to facilitate this process, a format that includes three components is used: (1) presentation by a facilitator of information and issues related to each key question, (2) a case study discussion that highlights some of the issues embedded within each question, and (3) semi-structured small group discussions and decision making. The workshops are organized such that these activities are provided for each key question.

Presentation and large group discussion led by a facilitator

Research[14] on school-based management suggests that teachers and other professionals cannot participate fully in decision making without some basic knowledge of the issues being discussed. Therefore, some instructor-led presentation is necessary. The content for the presentations is based on adult learning literature that suggests that any theoretical or research information must be clearly and explicitly tied to direct practice and daily work routines to ensure maximum relevance.[20] Discussion questions are used extensively throughout the presentation to facilitate participation and problem solving. Four components are addressed within each presentation. First, shared assumptions underlying a family-centered approach and the need for shared roles across team members are emphasized.[21] Second, the relevant rules and regulations from PL 99-457 are presented. If the state in which the workshop is being conducted has made relevant legislative or regulatory decisions, that information is included as well. Third, information about best practices related to the key question being discussed is presented so that participants will have at least some information about alternative courses of action and choices that could be made. Finally, the presentation includes a discussion of some of the issues that underlie any decisions that will be made. For example, the discussion might focus on ways in which assessing family needs could be perceived as intrusive by some families and helpful by others. Throughout the presentation, many alternative strategies, approaches, and techniques for working with families are provided, giving participants a chance to consider which ones might fit within their workplace. In addition, some information is provided about the change process itself, as a way of introducing the team-based, decision-making format.

Case study discussion

The primary goal of this activity is to provide participants an opportunity to apply and discuss issues in the context of a specific family and their interactions with an early intervention program. Although examples of issues and their application inevitably will emerge during the initial facilitator-led presentation, several case studies have been designed specifically to challenge professionals to consider how they might implement a family-centered philosophy in working with a particular family.[22]

Each case study is a relatively short (4 to 10 pages) description of a family and a particular set of issues faced by family members and the professional working in the program(s) serving the family. The case studies are based on the actual experiences of early interventionists in the field and represent the types of situations likely to be encountered by most early interventionists at some time in their work. The cases do not provide an answer to the conflicts faced by the professional(s) involved in the cases. Arriving at a solution or course of action for the professionals involved in the case is the objective of the discussion.

Case study discussion provides a structure for all participants in which exploration and application of the general principles of a family-centered approach are possible.[23,24] Although participants may wholeheartedly agree with the principles during the facilitator-led presentation and general discussion, attempts to apply the principles to the case study often result in an emerging awareness of personal biases and values as well as differences in interpreting the principles among participants (ie, team members) when it comes down to a specific case situation. Case study discussions are often quite lively, challenging the facilitator to keep discussions on track.

Team-based discussion and decision making

The activities described thus far may be conducted with a large group representing several teams or programs. Decision making, however, must occur at the team or program level. Thus the third activity involves teams in small group discussions and provides a framework for initial decision making related to each key question. The large group is divided into work teams for this activity. It is essential that small group participants include all of those individuals who work together or define themselves as a team in the provision of early intervention services. In addition, key administrators, supervisors, or other administrators should be present if at all possible.

A number of procedures have been suggested in the literature for using groups to obtain consensus on a topic. These include opinion surveys, focus groups, the nominal group process, and the Delphi technique.[25] The procedures differ in methods, assumptions, and level of formality, but all seek to obtain agreement among a group of individuals regarding needs, goals, or strategies.

In the present model, the challenge questions provide examples of how a family-centered approach might be operationalized, and they are used to help team members examine several dimensions of their program's practices and policies. Prior to the small group discussion, participants are given worksheets on which they indicate whether they think their program needs to change something in response to each of the challenge questions and rank each change in order of perceived importance. The group discussion then involves a sharing of individual rankings, with the goal being group consensus as to areas in which change is needed and a ranking of group priorities. Consensus is achieved, not through voting or taking an average of ratings, but rather by extended discussions until everyone agrees on the priority or course of action.

EFFECTIVE LEADERSHIP

The success of the workshop is highly dependent on the extent to which participants leave with a sense of authority over changes in program direction and confidence in the decisions they have made. The degree to which this occurs is, in part, dependent on certain qualities and skills of the workshop leader. The interactive nature of activities and the focus on empowering participants to make decisions require the leader to serve more as a consultant or facilitator than as an instructor. Although certain stylistic qualities may vary from one facilitator to another, research on consultation suggests several key attributes that are important to effective leadership.[26]

First, the facilitator must be knowledgeable about the issues being discussed. In this case, the facilitator must have some background and experience in working with young children with disabilities and their families. By sharing experiences and giving examples, the facilitator can bring to life many of the issues being discussed. Those experiences and examples must, however, relate to the experiences of the participants. The facilitator must also be familiar with PL 99-457, the regulations accompanying the law, and current or proposed rules and regulations for the state in which the workshop is being held. Furthermore, the facilitator needs to be familiar with major issues, trends, and procedures that have been discussed in the professional literature. Although the workshop is not designed to teach skills, the effectiveness of the leader in facilitating the discussion and decision-making process will depend in part on the participants' perception of the facilitator as a person who is knowledgeable about best practices and issues surrounding implementation of a family-centered approach.

Second, the facilitator must be able to engage participants in the workshop through use of effective questioning skills or by posing credible dilemmas to which the participants are expected to respond. The instructor's manual for the curriculum provides numerous examples of discussion questions. The facilitator will need to be able to ask these and other questions and respond to them in a fashion that encourages further participation and discussion.

Third, the facilitator must be flexible and be able to think on his or her feet. The activities will inevitably generate considerable discussion. Participants will give examples of families with whom they have worked that have posed challenges for them and will question the meaning of a family-centered approach relative to them. The facilitator must be able to accept all concerns as legitimate and be able to help participants see for themselves the relevance of a family-centered approach. This capability necessitates a nonjudgmental attitude, the ability to respond empathetically, and skills in engaging other participants in problem solving.

Finally, the facilitator must be able to set aside his or her own priorities and allow the participating teams to establish priorities for change as they see fit. This posture may be difficult in some cases, especially if the facilitator has strong ideas about what should be done; the facilitator, however, must realize that change is unlikely if priorities are imposed from the outside. Allowing teams to establish their own goals and priorities helps give teams ownership of the change process. If they succeed in areas they have identified, they may then move into other areas. Ultimately it is important for the facilitator to model for participants the same attitude and skills that participants should have in working with families.

• • •

How to implement family-centered services in the diverse communities that make up our country is a challenge and a goal for all of those involved in the current restructuring of human service programs.[27] For that goal to be accomplished, all persons involved in service provision will need to work together to define what they mean by family-centered practices and how that vision might be translated into day-to-day practices. Because family-centered principles can be operationalized in limitless ways, communities need strategies and opportunities to engage in systematic planning and goal setting. The model described in this article incorporates local team-based planning, consumer involvement, structured decision making, and principles of effective leadership as one way of facilitating that process. As programs continue to define and implement family-centered services in early intervention, this model and others should be systematically studied to determine the extent to which they result in meaningful and enduring change in early intervention programs and practices.

REFERENCES

1. Bailey DB, Buysse V, Edmondson R, Smith-Bonahue T. Creating family-centered services in early intervention: Perceptions of professionals in four states. *Except Children.* 1992;58:298–309.
2. Mahoney G, O'Sullivan P. Early intervention practices with families of children with handicaps. *Ment Retard.* 1990;28:169–176.
3. Mahoney G, O'Sullivan P, Fors S. The family practices of service providers for young handicapped children. *Inf Ment Health J.* 1989;10:75–83.
4. Brown J, Ritchie JA. Nurses' perceptions of parent and nurse roles in caring for hospitalized children. *Children's Health Care.* 1990;19:28–36.
5. Rushton CH. Family-centered care in the critical care setting: Myth or reality? *Children's Health Care.* 1990;19:68–77.
6. Bailey DB, Simeonsson RJ, Yoder D, Huntington GS. Preparing professionals to serve infants and toddlers with handicaps and their families: An integrative analysis across eight disciplines. *Except Children.* 1990;57:26–35.
7. Bailey DB, Palsha S, Simeonsson RJ. Professional skills, concerns, and perceived importance of work with families in early intervention. *Except Children.* 1991;58:156–165.
8. Shelton TL, Jeppson ES, Johnson BH. *Family-Centered Care for Children with Special Health Care Needs.* Washington, DC: Association for the Care of Children's Health; 1987.
9. Winton PJ. A systemic approach for planning inservice training related to Public Law 99-457. *Inf Young Children.* 1990;3:51–60.
10. Bailey DB, McWilliam PJ, Winton PJ, Simeonsson RJ. *Implementing Family-Centered Services in Early Intervention: A Team-Based Model for Change.* Chapel Hill, NC: Frank Porter Graham Child Development Center, University of North Carolina at Chapel Hill; 1991.
11. Fullan M. *The Meaning of Educational Change.* New York, NY: Teachers College Press; 1982.

12. Hall GE, Hord S. *Change in Schools: Facilitating the Process.* Albany, NY: State University of New York Press; 1987.
13. Havelock RG, Havelock MC. *Training for Change Agents.* Ann Arbor, Mich: University of Michigan; 1973.
14. David JL. Synthesis of research on school-based management. *Educational Leadership.* 1989;46:45–53.
15. Harrison CR, Killion JP, Mitchell JE. Site-based management: The realities of implementation. *Educational Leadership.* 1989;46:55–58.
16. Peck CA, Killen CC, Baumgart D. Increasing implementation of special education instruction in mainstream preschools: Direct and generalized effects of nondirective consultation. *J Appl Behav Anal.* 1989;22:197–210.
17. Burke EM. Citizen participation strategies. *J Am Inst Planning.* 1968;34:287–294.
18. Katan J, Prager E. Consumer and worker participation in agency-level decision-making: Some considerations of their linkages. *Admin Social Work.* 1986;10:79–88.
19. Bailey DB, Buysse V, Smith-Bonahue T, Elam J. The effects and perceptions of family involvement in program decisions about family-centered practices. *Eval Program Planning.* 1992;15:23–32.
20. Knowles MS. *The Adult Learner.* Houston, Tex: Gulf; 1984.
21. McCollum JA, Thorp EK. Training of infant specialists: A look to the future. *Inf Young Children.* 1988;1:55–65.
22. McWilliam PJ. *The Families We Serve: Case Studies in Early Intervention.* Chapel Hill, NC: Frank Porter Graham Child Development Center, University of North Carolina at Chapel Hill; 1991.
23. Graham PT, Cline PC. The case method: A basic teaching approach. *Theory Into Practice.* 1980;19:112–116.
24. Kreps GL, Lederman LC. Using the case method in organizational communication education: Developing students' insight, knowledge, and creativity through experience-based learning and systematic debriefing. *Communication Ed.* 1985;34:358–364.
25. Zemke R, Kramlinger T. *Figuring Things Out: A Trainer's Guide to Needs and Task Analysis.* Reading, Mass: Addison-Wesley; 1987.
26. Coleman PP, Buysse V, Scalise-Smith DL, Schulte AC. Consultation: Applications to early intervention. *Inf Young Children.* 1991;4:1–6.
27. Farrow F. Services to families: The view from the states. *Fam Society.* 1991;72:268–275.

Appendix

Key questions about family-centered practices in early intervention

What is our philosophy about working with families?

- Is a family focus central to our program philosophy and shared by all team members?
- Have families been invited to collaborate in the development of our program philosophy?
- Are our interactions with families positive?
- Do we respect family diversity in beliefs, values, and coping styles?
- Are our services flexible enough to meet individual family needs?
- Does our IFSP process recognize and support informal support systems?
- Do we allow families to refuse help?

How will we involve families in child assessment?

- Are we complying with all PL 99-457 regulations regarding child assessment?
- Do we try to determine family preferences about the purpose and format of child assessment, as well as their wish to be involved?
- Do we convey assessment information in a sensitive and jargon-free fashion?
- Does the family's perception of the child's needs determine the focus of child assessment?
- Do we listen to the family's preferences in determining settings, times, and parent roles in child assessment?
- Do we address children's strengths in the assessment process?
- Do we validate or check the results of our assessment activities against the views of families?

How will we identify family needs and strengths?

- Are we complying with all PL 99-457 regulations regarding family assessment?
- Do parents know that we are responsive to family needs?
- Do we try to determine family preferences regarding family assessment?
- Have we agreed on a flexible model and alternative procedures for assessing family needs and strengths?
- Is family assessment recognized as part of each team member's role?
- Does each team member have the skills needed to communicate effectively with families?

How will we involve families in team meetings and decision making?

- Are we complying with all PL 99-457 regulations regarding the team and family participation on it?
- Do we try to determine family preferences regarding their role on the team?
- Do families determine team membership?
- Do we employ strategies to make sure that families feel comfortable participating in team meetings?
- Do we function as a team or as individual specialists?
- Do we hold our meetings in settings and times convenient to the family?
- Do we respect parents' decisions even if professionals disagree?

What will be the format of an IFSP or IEP?

- Are we complying with all PL 99-457 regulations regarding the IFSP or IEP document?
- Do we try to determine family preferences regarding their role in developing or writing the IFSP?
- Have we agreed on an IFSP format that will work for us?
- Do we write goals using words that are acceptable and understandable for families?

How will we implement the IFSP and provide case management services?

- Are we complying with all PL 99-457 regulations regarding service provision and case management?
- Do we try to determine family preferences regarding their role in case management and service coordination?
- Have we decided who will serve as case managers?
- Have we determined the skills and training that will be needed by case managers?

Negotiation and problem-solving strategies: Collaboration between families and professionals

Patricia Brandt, PhD
Associate Professor
Department of Parent and Child Nursing
University of Washington School of Nursing
Seattle, Washington

PROFESSIONALS are legislated by Part H of the Individuals with Disabilities Education Act Amendment of 1991 to involve families in the development of the Individualized Family Service Plan (IFSP) and in service coordination.[1] The guidelines for an IFSP require that the family's resources, priorities, and concerns be included and that outcomes be relevant for the child and the family. Through service coordination, families are assisted in identifying service providers and in accessing agency cooperation for the delivery of services. The family and professional are encouraged to collaborate during these activities.[2–4] This article describes negotiation and problem-solving strategies and their value for promoting collaboration between the family and professional.

What is the meaning of the word *collaboration*? Webster's dictionary defines collaboration as "to cooperate with or work jointly with others in an endeavor." The following is a summary of characteristics that typify collaboration as found in the literature on parent-professional relationships[5–7]:

- specified joint rights and responsibilities
- mutually accessible and responsible collaboration
- mutual respect for skills and knowledge
- mutually understood communication
- mutually agreed-upon goals
- joint planning and decision making
- joint follow-through of solutions, evaluation, and revisions

How do negotiation and problem-solving strategies contribute to collaboration? Negotiation and problem-solving strategies are important for implementing a collaborative relationship because these strategies enhance the definition of rights and responsibilities, goal setting, joint planning, decision making, and follow-through of solutions. Negotiation is defined as a strategy that resolves issues between two or more people primarily through discussion, bargaining, and compromise.[8,9] Problem solving is a strategy that involves defining concern(s), exploring goal(s) and concern(s), and determining and acting on solutions.[10] The product of

Preparation of this manuscript was partially supported by a Children and Adolescents with Special Health Care Needs Training grant from the Bureau of Maternal and Child Health, Department of Health and Human Services (grant 909). The contents are in no way the responsibility of the Department of Health and Human Services.

Inf Young Children 1993; 5(4): 78–84

these two strategies is a contract that explicitly defines the goal(s), solution(s), responsibilities, and reinforcers for the progress and outcomes achieved. Family members and professionals need to have skills in problem solving and negotiation for collaboration to be effective during the IFSP and service coordination activities.[11,12]

THE PROBLEM-SOLVING STRATEGY

Problem solving consists of four phases: definition of the concern(s), generation of alternative solutions, decision making, and planning the implementation.[10] Through a problem-solving approach, IFSP and service coordination activities are promoted by identifying the family's concerns and the related services that best match the child's and family's particular needs. A problem-solving approach provides a format for naturally progressing from one step to the next and, thus, decreases the likelihood of getting stuck in one of the steps or overwhelmed with complex and potentially conflicting issues. Throughout problem solving, the professional participates by guiding the family members through each phase with explanations and demonstrations as needed.

The first phase of problem solving, definition of the concern, is dominated by two activities.[10] First, each family member expresses a viewpoint of what the major concern is, and other family members and the professional(s) verify that they understand the identified concern or request further explanation. The second activity involves a discussion of each concern within a previously agreed-upon time limit. All concerns are then prioritized.[10] During the definition phase, it is essential for the professional to ensure that each concern is clearly defined and understood. The perspective of each family member is directly obtained whenever possible. Children are encouraged to participate as their communication skills permit. If a family member is not present or has limited verbal skills, other members are asked, for example, "What would Johnny say was the major issue he'd like us to deal with in our meeting today?"

The second phase of a problem-solving strategy is the generation of solutions.[10] Each family member has a turn in which he or she volunteers ideas toward resolving the agreed-upon major concern. During this phase each member is encouraged to be involved, to be creative, and not to be governed by the solutions traditionally used. A critique occurs only after all ideas are generated. When a family member finds it difficult to participate in solution generation, the professional and/or other family members can encourage that person to begin with ideas of what has worked well in the past, to expand on these past solutions, and then to generate new solutions. If a member continues to have difficulty generating solutions, a discussion of the roadblocks should be held with ways for overcoming these outlined.[8,9] Examples of perceived roadblocks could be ongoing conflict between two family members and a lack of funds for transportation.

During the third phase of problem solving, decision making, the advantages and disadvantages of solutions generated are discussed by the family and are rated by each member.[10] Negotiation is often used during this phase to form a compromise that maximizes short- and long-term advantages and considers each family member and the family as a unit. Those solutions found to have major disadvantages or significant negative consequences need to be omitted at this time. An important role of the professional during this phase is to encourage each member to go beyond statements such as "That'll never work for me," "It's OK," and "I don't know" by encouraging the translation of statements such as these into opinions. If a family member is given opportunities to express his or her beliefs and refuses to explain or expand, the professional and other family members should respect that person's refusal at the time and provide other chances during the session or, if possible, at another meeting.

The fourth and final phase of a problem-solving strategy is planning the implementation.[10] The family delineates what specific actions will be taken to implement the solutions. Each family member and the professional, as appropriate to the concern and solutions identified, determines who will be responsible for each action. Ways for monitoring progress, reinforcing each other, and renegotiating solutions are also outlined. Trouble-shooting approaches for problems that arise during implementation also need to be determined during this phase. A written contract that outlines the implementation plan is used as a summary of the collaborative work. A contract acts as a vehicle for clarifying issues that evolve and ensures that each person has a similar memory of the agreement. When completing the contract, the professional and family are given another opportunity to ensure that their plan is clear and understandable to those involved. Although a written contract needs to be developed with all families, a verbal report of the implementation of the contract's activities may be preferable for some families rather than keeping a log of each activity performed. Families who do not have highly conflictual interactions may prefer verbal monitoring of progress and reporting of outcomes. As long as the family members who are involved in the plan share in the responsibility of tracking and reporting progress, a verbal method appears effective. If young children are involved, charts with stars are helpful so that the children are able to visualize progress and success. A follow-up meeting should always be planned to determine progress and to renegotiate alternative solutions because about one of five solutions has been found to need renegotiation.[13]

THE NEGOTIATION STRATEGY

Negotiation ensures that effective decision making occurs during IFSP and service coordination activities. Negotiation enhances compromise and conflict resolution among family members and ensures that the child's perspective and needs are important considerations in the concerns and the solutions generated.[11,14] When the family has been a team member throughout the assessment and early intervention activities, and when a family-focused approach has been used, a focus on the child as well as on relevant needs of other family members is more likely to evolve during the problem-solving phases.[15–18]

When disagreement occurs during the IFSP or service coordination activities, the negotiation strategy offers promise for resolving conflicts in a positive and constructive context.[8–10] To negotiate a compromise, one should start with solutions rated with a few advantages by at least two of those involved in the disagreement. Each person should be directed toward the overall goal, and compatible, common interests in the solution need to be identified. In addition, conflicting interests need to be made explicit.

Agreements that are satisfactory to the family are more likely to be attained during negotiation when members are separated from the problem, when mutual interests and gains are accentuated, and when objective criteria are used to evaluate the solutions generated.[9] If feelings arise during negotiation, they need to be acknowledged in an understanding and time-limited manner. A reactive stance and discounting and blaming comments, however, are not conducive to negotiation and thus need to be avoided during these discussions or stopped if they occur. Ground rules need to be formulated before brainstorming of solutions so that the sharing of ideas occurs in a safe environment. A win-win orientation also needs to be promoted so that mutual interests and gains for all are the predominant attitudes. Before solutions are evaluated and prioritized, concrete, fair, and appropriate criteria need to be selected. Throughout the negotiation process, family members should be urged to use the encouraging and positive reinforcing approaches that they typically use with each other. The professional also needs verbally to recognize each member's attempts at idea generation and compromise.

Throughout the negotiation process, the professional's multipositional orientation toward the family ensures that the interests of each family member are known and understood and that the child's physical and psychosocial needs are addressed adequately.[19,20] Decisions about concerns or solutions should not be interpreted by the family as being due to the alignment of the professional with a particular family member but should be perceived as a compromise that is beneficial to the family. The professional can be instrumental in enabling the expansion of existing options by giving novel approaches, perhaps those used by other families in similar situations, so that various possibilities are considered.

When a compromise is still difficult for a particular family member, negotiation is more likely to move forward when each member identifies his or her bottom line. The member who cannot agree to the identified solutions is asked to generate a solution that will promote compromise and acknowledge the bottom line of the others.[8–10] The professional also needs to assess whether abuse or safety issues may be interfering in a member's participation during problem solving and/or negotiation. Appropriate resources and necessary agencies need to be contacted as required by law or as dictated by professional ethics. If a potential abuse situation is identified, problem-solving and negotiation strategies may need to be halted temporarily or perhaps used with individual family members rather than with the family as a group.

COMMUNICATION SKILLS FOR PROBLEM SOLVING AND NEGOTIATION

Family members and professionals who collaborate with each other benefit from having the communication skills needed for successful problem solving and negotiation. Robin and Foster[10] found that negative communication behaviors distracted and interfered with problem-solving discussions. Examples of problematic communications are verbal behaviors such as lecturing or making defensive statements and nonverbal behaviors such as fidgeting or having minimal eye contact. Before mutually acceptable solutions can be obtained during a problem-solving skills training intervention, new behaviors need to be learned. Problematic behaviors will then be markedly diminished.[10]

In a study of the IFSP process, good communication skills were identified as central to effective collaboration by both professionals and parents.[3] Verbal communication skills that are especially valuable for families and professionals during negotiation and problem solving are listening or attending to the message by paraphrasing, clarifying, and checking perceptions; reflecting feelings, experience, and content; leading or focusing skills and encouraging discussion; and informing by giving valid information based on experience, using "I" statements, and being clear and brief.[21] Verbal communication skills need to be accompanied by such nonverbal skills as using a neutral tone of voice, sitting relaxed, and using eye contact.

For effective problem solving and negotiation to occur, communication skills need to be exercised in the context of a professional-family relationship that is oriented to action. According to Brammar's[21] helping model, change occurs as a result of the professional and family working together during two phases. During phase 1, the focus is building the relationship; in phase 2, action occurs. The major components of the building relationship phase are as follows:

- convening at a time and in a setting that is convenient for the significant family members;
- clarifying the family's overall concerns and obtaining the comprehensive and relevant information associated with the concerns (professionals and family members share beliefs about collaboration; confidentiality and policies of the agency are explained);

- structuring, with overall goals being described by the family; timeliness, duration, frequency, cost, and location of possible services are explained by the professional;
- acknowledging and identifying roles and functions of the relationships in the context of the family's resources; the professional's functions and abilities are defined.

In addition to the listening, reflecting, learning, and informing skills needed by both family members and professionals during phase 1, the professional needs to use summarizing, interpreting, and positive confronting skills, which serve to interrupt interfering behavior, to point out discrepancies, and to model alternatives while the relationship is being built.

The helping model outlined by Brammar[21] incorporates problem solving and negotiation as action components central to phase 2 activities. During phase 2, the professional and family work together toward the desired outcomes. If communication skills need to be strengthened to progress with the work of phase 2, skills training occurs at this time. The professional on the team, no matter what his or her discipline, needs to communicate effectively and to be skilled in problem solving and negotiation. One of the team members may have the expertise to provide the interpersonal skills development needed by a professional or family, or the team may need to consult with or refer to other resources. During the early part of the action phase, families may feel that so much has been accomplished that they terminate prematurely, before acting on solutions. For example, after the work involved in clearly defining the major concern, providing comprehensive information about the concern, and generating ideas toward solutions, some families cancel appointments or terminate. Thus it is essential that the collaborative activities started while the relationship is being built continue throughout the action phase. Feelings of discouragement, frustration, and fatigue need to be identified and ways to address these feelings discovered jointly.

Many factors may interfere with progress during the action phase. During phase 1, sufficient attention to building a collaborative relationship may not have occurred, or phase 2 may have moved too quickly for sufficient collection and synthesis of information. Other factors also need to be considered if collaborative work is unsuccessful. The professional involved may not have the necessary interpersonal, problem-solving, or negotiation skills.[10,19,22] The family's socioeconomic and cultural/ethnic backgrounds may not have been adequately considered during the relationship building or action phases.[23] The beliefs and attitudes of the professional and/or family members may also be impeding progress.

Problematic expectations or beliefs of family members and the professional play a significant role in delaying progress or interfering in collaborative relationships. Beliefs that promote collaboration are described by Dunst et al[6] as empowerment and enabling. Empowerment is equated with working with families so that they maintain or acquire a sense of control over their family life and believe that the positive changes that occur are a result of their own strengths, abilities, and actions. Enabling provides ways for families to demonstrate their present abilities and competencies while acquiring new skills needed for problem solving and negotiation.

What beliefs encourage empowering and enabling during collaboration? Examples of beliefs of professionals that promote collaboration are as follows[2–6]:

- Parents are experts about their own child.
- Parents' time and work are as important as professionals' time and work.
- Parents are resources with abilities and strengths; they are not adversaries.
- Difficulties during collaborative work are influenced by the interaction of family members as well as the agencies and professionals.
- The family is responsible for having their concerns met; the professional's role is one that provides accountable, accessible services appropriate to the family's defined concerns.

Examples of enabling and empowering beliefs of parents that promote collaborative work with professionals include the following[2–6]:

- Parents are equal partners with professionals and have the primary responsibility for the child's care.
- Parents communicate their needs and their child's needs to professionals accurately and promptly.
- Past negative experiences with professionals or agencies do not interfere in current working relationships.
- Commitments are followed through, and changes are communicated to professionals at an appropriate time.
- Parents' expectations of the professional, their child, and themselves are realistic.

When continued conflict occurs or when collaboration does not proceed, consultation with a team member or outside resource with expertise in counseling and cognitive strategies would be valuable. Cognitive restructuring strategies have been found to be useful for altering or replacing negative perceptions that interfere in positive communication and problem solving.[10] Offering alternative, positive ways of viewing a situation and understanding the connections among thoughts, feelings, and behaviors contribute to family members relating positively to each other and to the level of collaboration achieved between the professional and the family. Communication skills training programs have been developed and are a valuable resource for an early intervention team that incorporates family-centered practices.[24–26]

• • •

The professional is able to focus on the family agenda and to capitalize on the family's strengths when he or she uses problem-solving and negotiation strategies.

Professionals are also more likely not to be a major stress in the family's life if the family and professional are engaged in collaborative endeavors.[27] Evidence from research indicates that outcomes are more positive when interventions meet family needs and have a family-centered approach.[5,18] Strong decision-making abilities of parents have also been found to be related to better child outcomes.[28]

Throughout the collaborative process, each family member's adaptation to the diagnosis and management of the child's condition should be explicitly acknowledged by the family members and the professional. A family member may be more ready to participate in collaborative endeavors and help-seeking if he or she is experiencing outward focusing rather than an impact, denial, or grief phase.[27,29] Continual acknowledgment of each other's contributions and strengths will enhance ongoing relationship building and actions toward implementing solutions that are family centered.

REFERENCES

1. Rule-making for early intervention programs for infants and toddlers with disabilities. *Federal Register.* May 1, 1992;57:18996, 19003, 19004.
2. Leadership Development for Nurses in Early Intervention Project. *National Standards of Nursing Practice for Early Intervention Services.* Lexington, Ky: Division of Parent-Child Nursing, University of Kentucky; 1991.
3. DeGangi G, Royun C, Wietlisbach S. How to examine the individualized family service plan process: preliminary findings and a procedural guide. *Infants Young Child.* 1992;5:42–56.
4. Bailey DB. Collaborative goal-setting with families: resolving differences in values and priorities for services. *Top Early Child Spec Educ.* 1987;7:59–71.
5. Dunst CJ, Trivette CM, Davis M, Cornwell J. Enabling and empowering families of children with health impairments. *Child Health Care.* 1988;17:71–81.
6. Dunst C, Trivette C, Angela D. *Enabling and Empowering Families: Principles and Guidelines for Practice.* Cambridge, Mass: Brookline; 1988.
7. Turnbull AP, Turnbull HR. *Families, Professionals and Exceptionality.* Columbus, Ohio: Merrill; 1986.
8. Northwest Mediation Service. *Mediation Skills for Managers.* Bellevue, Wash: Northwest Mediation Service; 1991.
9. Fisher R, Ury W. *Getting to Yes: Negotiating Agreement without Giving In.* New York, NY: Viking; 1981.
10. Robin A, Foster S. *Negotiating Parent-Adolescent Conflict.* New York, NY: Guilford; 1989.
11. Bailey D, McWilliam P, Winton P. Building family centered practices in early intervention: a team based model for change. *Infants Young Child.* 1992;5:73–82.
12. McGonigel M, Garland C. The individualized family service plan and the early intervention team: team and family issues and recommended practices. *Infants Young Child.* 1988;1:10–21.
13. Foster SL. *Family Conflict Management Skills Training and Generalization Procedures.* Stony Brook, NY: State University of New York; 1978. Thesis.

14. Kohnke MF. *Advocacy: Risk and Reality.* St Louis, Mo: Mosby; 1982.
15. Bailey D, Simeonsson R. *Family Assessment in Early Intervention.* Columbus, Ohio: Merrill; 1988.
16. Wasik B, Bryant D, Lyons C. *Home Visiting: Procedures for Helping Families.* Newbury Park, Calif: Sage; 1990.
17. Barber PA, Turnbull AP, Behr SK, Kerns GM. A family systems perspective in early childhood special education. In: Odom S, Karnes M, eds. *Early Intervention for Infants and Children with Handicaps.* Baltimore, Md: Brookes; 1988.
18. Sloman L, Konstantareas M. Why families of children with biological deficits require a systems approach. *Fam Process.* 1990;29:417–429.
19. Wright L, Leahey M. *Families and Chronic Illness.* Springhouse, Pa: Springhouse; 1987.
20. Godfrey A. Providing health services to facilitate benefit from early intervention: a model. *Infants Young Child.* 1991;4:47–55.
21. Brammar L. *The Helping Relationship: Process and Skills.* Englewood Cliffs, NJ: Prentice-Hall; 1988.
22. Morse J. Negotiating commitment and involvement in the nurse-patient relationship. *J Adv Nurs.* 1991; 16:455–468.
23. Anderson P, Fenichel E. *Serving Culturally Diverse Families of Infants and Toddlers with Disabilities.* Washington, DC: National Center for Clinical Infant Programs; 1989.
24. Dinkmeyer D, McKay G. *Systematic Training for Effective Parenting.* Circle Pines, Minn: American Guidance Service; 1990.
25. Faber A, Mazlish E. *How To Talk so Kids Will Listen.* New York, NY: Negotiation Institute; 1980.
26. Carkhuff RR, Anthony WA. *The Skills of Helping.* Amherst, MA: Human Resource Development Press; 1986.
27. Thomas RB. The struggle for control between families and health care providers when a child has complex health care needs. *Zero Three.* 1988;15–18.
28. Deaton A. Adaptive noncompliance in pediatric asthma, parents as expert. *J Pediatr Psychol.* 1985;11:1–13.
29. Roberts S. Social support and help seeking: review of the literature. *Adv Nurs Sci.* 1988;10:1–11.

Family administered neonatal activities: An adaptation for parents of infants born with Down syndrome

Ida Anne Cardone, PhD
Clinical Psychologist

Linda Gilkerson, PhD
Infant Care Program
Department of Pediatrics
Evanston Hospital
Evanston, Illinois

I think "coming to terms" means seeing the child for him or herself—a unique person with his (her) own special problems and special qualities.[1(p28)]

THE PROCESS OF "coming to terms" is one of the ongoing challenges of parenthood. Brazelton[2] asserts that during pregnancy, parents prepare themselves for two infants: the hoped for, healthy infant and the infant with disabilities. This preparatory process mobilizes energy that then helps parents adapt to the infant who is born to them.

The unexpected birth of an infant with Down syndrome can be experienced as a shattering event to parents in the moments, hours, and days after the birth of their son or daughter. In reports of the intensity of distress at 10 developmental crisis points, Wikler and coworkers[3] found that the time of diagnosis was the most distressful period for families. In the past, the time of diagnosis for infants with Down syndrome ranged from the first week to the first year and after.[4] Current pediatric practice recommends informing parents of the clinical signs of Down syndrome as soon as they are evident, which is often very shortly after delivery, even though the formal diagnosis through chromosomal analysis may not be made for 72 hours. Thus, the vast majority of families are informed about the possibility or reality of Down syndrome in the hospital.[5]

Early diagnosis presents physicians, nurses, and other hospital-based family support personnel with a unique opportunity and a poignant challenge. During this time when families are most deeply affected, professionals are also experiencing acute emotional reactions. Parents have reported a range of responses from health care professionals. Some individuals are understanding, empathic, informative, and truly helpful, while others are less able to offer positive assistance because of their own sadness, insecurity, or limited knowledge of Down syndrome.[6] Regardless of the nature of the parent–professional interaction, parents remember these initial experiences years later. Noting the "freshness of their memories of early

The authors thank the families for teaching us what is needed and Sheila Heibein and Kristine Weisenberger for sharing their rich experience and wise counsel. Copies of the manual, A Hospital-Based, Multidisciplinary Approach to the Unexpected Delivery of an Infant with Down Syndrome *can be obtained from I. Cardone, Department of Pediatrics, Evanston Hospital, 2650 Ridge Avenue, Evanston, IL 60201.*

Inf Young Children 1992; 5(1): 40–48

impact,"[5(p394)] Gath reports that families vividly recalled these contacts. Moreover, Gath found that "sometimes fine details are recounted almost word for word, particularly when the event was very painful."[5(p394)]

FAMILY ADMINISTERED NEONATAL ACTIVITIES

This article describes an approach that has been helpful in supporting families during the immediate postpartum hospital stay, a time when, as one father stated, professionals have a true opportunity to "minister to people's needs." This approach is a modification of the Family Administered Neonatal Activities (FANA),[7,8] which is a specialized adaptation of the Neonatal Behavioral Assessment Scale (NBAS).[9] The FANA guides parents in eliciting behaviors from their newborn within the context of a structured process that integrates the practices of short-term, focused, psychodynamic interviewing with the principles of an empowerment model. The NBAS was chosen as the ideal tool around which to develop a clinical intervention because it provides a systematic method for observing and eliciting the behavioral capacities of the newborn. The primary goals of the FANA are

- to promote a sense of mastery over events of pregnancy, labor, and delivery;
- to affirm and enhance parental capacities to observe and engage their infant; and
- to provide a forum for the integration of initial parental perceptions and expectations with the infant's present behavior.

The FANA intervention takes place on the second day postpartum in the mother's room with mother, father, and infant present. The FANA, which takes about 40 to 50 minutes, is routinely offered to all first-time families and to families referred by the attending obstetrician, pediatrician, or primary nurse. The reasons for referral are multiple, including parental fear of handling their infant, resurgence of grief due to prior perinatal loss, or an especially difficult labor and delivery. The FANA can serve as a source of support to affirm already existing parental strengths and resources, as an intervention when events of the near history complicate parental perception of and interaction with the infant, or as an assessment when questions arise as to the capacity of the family to care for the child at home.

The FANA process includes three phases: phase I: parent perception interview, phase II: NBAS application, and phase III: integrative summary. The theoretical framework and clinical model are presented in detail in Cardone and Gilkerson.[7,8] The following paragraphs present a brief description of each phase.

Phase I: Parent perception interview

Prior to meeting with the families, the facilitator reads the mother's and infant's chart to learn about parental history, health concerns, and infant status. The family contact portion of the FANA begins with the parent perception interview. This interview includes a greeting and a 10 to 15 minute conversation with the parents about four areas: (1) their personal well-being, (2) their labor and delivery experience, (3) the infant's name and the historical significance of the name, and (4) their observations and perceptions of the infant. The questions asked of each parent are: How are you? How was your labor and delivery? What is your infant's name? Was he or she named after someone special? What have you noticed about your infant so far? The facilitator is trained not to normalize the experience (ie, "All new mothers feel that way"); not to prematurely reassure (ie, "You'll feel better soon"); or at this point, not to teach new information. The facilitator listens empathetically, encourages elaboration and expression of feelings, and acknowledges questions and concerns. This phase sets a tone of emotional sensitivity, responsiveness, and reciprocity. It also provides the first of many opportunities to acknowledge and affirm already existing parental competencies (ie, "You've noticed so much about your infant already. Let's see what else she has to tell us about herself.")

Phase II: NBAS application

Next, with the support and guidance of the facilitator, the parents engage in a hands-on exploration of their newborn's behavior. The NBAS application phase uses 28 items selected for the NBAS. Depending on the infant's state, the activities include habituation, orientation, selected reflexes, and consolability. The facilitator is trained to invite, encourage, guide, and, when needed, assist families in carrying out these activities themselves. Rather than interpreting the newborn to the family, the facilitator encourages parents to discover and share their own interpretations of their infant's behavior. Information on infant behavior is provided if it is relevant to a parental observation or concern. In this stage, the infant has the opportunity to speak for himself or herself through the language of newborn behavior.

Phase III: Integrative summary

During the integrative summary, the family is guided in reflecting on what they have just seen and in integrating these observations with their comments in the initial parental perception interview. After a brief summary, the facilitator asks: "How do you feel about what we just did together? What did you see that you expected to see? What did you see that surprised you? Let's think about what the next few weeks may bring as you care for your infant at home." More often than not, the concrete interactive experience with their newborn affirms the initial parental observations. At times, when the infant's behavior challenges parental perceptions, the FANA offers a unique opportunity for parents to recalibrate their first impressions. For example, a father wept as he described his trauma at witnessing the forceps delivery of his son: "Look at him. He's so flimsy. How could anyone born like that be well." During the NBAS application, the father saw his very robust son reflexively walk and crawl. "He's not flimsy at all," the father commented during the integrative summary.

FACILITATOR TRAINING

FANA facilitators receive intensive training beyond NBAS reliability. The training includes family systems and object relations theory as well as multiple observations and supervised hands-on experience. Prerequisites to FANA training include an advanced degree in child development, social work, psychology, early childhood special education, or a related field and a minimum of 3 years working with infants and families. These are formidable requirements, but the quality of the FANA experience depends on the facilitator's ability to maintain a sensitive balance of clinical and developmental skills within a relationship characterized by respect and reciprocity.

THE MODIFIED FANA PROCESS

For families of infants with Down syndrome, the modified FANA is designed as an initial, hospital-based experience to facilitate parental efforts at adjustment and to serve as a transitional link to the community. This application of the FANA was developed after multiple clinical experiences with families who had unexpectedly delivered an infant with Down syndrome. It was recognized early on that a large component of effective support of parents during the newborn period related to grief counseling. In the absence of acknowledgement of the sorrow, rage, and helplessness that sometimes occur with the birth, additional support and intervention were not fruitful. Thus, the FANA process was adapted to extend the first phase into two contacts to allow families more time to begin to process the powerful emotions accompanying the birth and to receive support as they reach out to family and friends. Engaging the families with their infant through the NBAS application occurs on the third contact. While the primary experience with this modification of the FANA has been for families of infants with Down syndrome, the general principles may also apply to infants born with congenital physical differences such as limb deformities, cleft lip and palate, and birthmarks.

Goals of the modified FANA

The FANA intervention for parents of newborns with Down syndrome has three primary goals:

1. to recognize and acknowledge the parents' emotional responses to the birth of their infant,
2. to facilitate the efforts of parents to reach out to family members and friends at a time when they need support but simultaneously may be apprehensive or ambivalent about making contact, and
3. to provide an opportunity for parents to observe and interact with their infant in order to highlight
   - the infant's uniqueness,
   - the parental capacity for observation, and
   - the special challenges and rewards of interaction with an infant with Down syndrome.

Implementation of the process

The FANA process is implemented through a series of visits with parents occurring during the postpartum stay.

Visit 1: Parental response to the birth and perceptions of the infant

The initial contact takes place in the first 24 hours after birth. The timing of this visit is decided in collaboration with the family's primary nurse. This visit provides an opportunity for parents to share their emotional responses to the birth of their infant as well as their initial perceptions of the infant.

In those first, important introductory moments, the facilitator must convey several messages. First, there must be a clear, gentle acknowledgment of the birth in the context of acceptance for whatever feelings the parents bring to this moment. For example, "I've talked to your nurse; I know there's a strong possibility your infant has Down syndrome. You must have been through a lot in these last 24 hours. What's it been like for you?" The facilitator must be ready to see a broad range of emotions, including anger, grief, fear, confusion, and, even at this early moment, acceptance. Assumptions cannot be made about what to expect, but one can be reasonably certain that feelings will be extremely heightened.

Second, the facilitator must provide a steadying and supportive presence. Are the parents tired? Are they comfortable? Has a cot been provided for the father if he wishes to spend a night in the hospital? Anxieties and needs must be acknowledged at the same time as efforts at soothing prevail.

Third, the facilitator must convey a sense of certainty of purpose. Clinical experience teaches that parents need to know that the service provider is comfortable in that role and knows the hospital system. Parents also need to feel that they are in good hands at a time when they may feel on very tentative ground and have a sense that time is standing still. The facilitator should alert the parents to what is going to happen next: "I would like to see you early tomorrow (or later today). You have so much to say. We'll talk more. I'll see you one more time after that before you go home and we will engage [infant's name] together." One father remarked, 'She [the facilitator] went right into action. It gave us the feeling that there was some kind of rhyme or reason to this thing."

Finally, the facilitator must convey a sense of interest in the newborn, at a time when the parents may not yet know how they feel about their infant or what they may hear from family and friends. The facilitator may say, "So tell me what you've noticed about your newborn so far." In those first moments the facilitator is acutely aware that parents are dealing simultaneously with the loss of a wished-for child while making those first furtive attempts at accepting and relating to the reality of their newborn—a newborn who has preemptive needs for care and affection regardless of the presence of Down syndrome.[10]

Counter-transferential issues in this work can be enormously challenging. It is simply easier to hear some things more than others. One of the greatest professional challenges is to hear: "I wish he were dead. What can we do to be sure he dies." This parental statement is extreme but is a measure of the anguish with which a family is living. In this circumstance, the facilitator must rely on the support of colleagues on the team. There must be an open, accepting forum to share the emotion evoked through the work and to develop strategies for maintaining perspective at a time when the facilitator's role is complex and challenging. This role is to allow full emotional expression for the parents—accepting them just where they are in relation to the infant—while maintaining a confident posture and positive regard for the infant.

Mrs Brown is a 30-year-old who has a 4-year-old son and a newborn daughter with Down syndrome. When the facilitator entered the room, the infant was draped across her mother's lap, not cradled or touched. As Mrs Brown talked about her feelings, she described her newborn as an "it." She felt that this was a "situation" rather than an infant. She described the "it" as floppy, as an "old woman who felt like a marshmallow"; this was "someone who can't suck, who drools, and who won't wake up." Mrs Brown spent 20 minutes of the initial interview crying, poignantly describing her intense ambivalence regarding this infant, that is, not wanting her but feeling terrified whenever the baby was not near her.

At very early times like this, the facilitator may hear statements such as "He looks like an alien, look at him, my alien." Or, from a father, "The labor and delivery was so easy, and then this . . ." and "There goes my concert pianist." There are also expressions of guilt and self-blame. "What could I have done wrong. I think it was the flu I had during my first trimester," or "I told my cousin I shouldn't be eating Thai food in my fifth month." The facilitator acknowledges that these are very painful feelings to be living with. In this first visit, parents cannot be reassured. They are typically not interested in the facts at this point. Fathers very often find it hard to share their feelings during the initial interview. It is not unusual to see a father sitting silently, his head in his hands. "We were two crushed people," one father remembered. "They just let us commiserate for a while."

Visit 2: Exploration of parental initiative to announce the birth

In this visit, which usually lasts at least 30 minutes, there is an effort to examine more fully what the parents understand about Down syndrome and to begin to help them reach out to their world beyond the hospital. Typical questions explore what the parents will say to family and friends and how they will say it. The facilitator might begin by asking, "Who have you told about the birth of your baby?"

Mrs Foley, a first-time parent, asked, "How will I tell my mother?" The facilitator suggested that alternatives be explored and helped her try out different scenarios. Mrs Foley said, "I might say that my child is mentally retarded, but that would feel awful." The facilitator wondered what might feel better. Mrs Foley thought that it would feel better to simply say, "My baby has Down syndrome." She added, "I'll tell her my baby won't learn as fast as other children. She will probably wonder if her grandchild will be able to know her and love her and kiss her. Then what can I say?" The facilitator replied that a child with Down syndrome can be as lovable and as stubborn as any other child.

At the time of the second visit, parents may ask about their child's developmental needs. For example, one father wanted to know if his child would have to be institutionalized. The facilitator must be knowledgeable about both the developmental range and educational needs of children with Down syndrome and the services that are available in the community. At this time, families are advised that no predictions can be made now about the future, but that their child *will* grow and develop and that they will too, right along with their child.

At the time of the second visit, many families are ready for contact with an outreach parent from a local Down syndrome association. For many parents this contact can be quite important because it assures them that others have faced a similar situation and made it through. Outreach parents may visit the family as long as needed after discharge. Information about early intervention may be presented by the staff, but outreach parents are also excellent sources of information about community resources.

Visit 3: Parental observation of and interaction with their infant

During the third visit, usually held on the second day postpartum near the time of discharge, the focus is on the infant and the parents together. The facilitator introduces the NBAS application and follows with the integrative summary.

The facilitator adapts the beginning of the NBAS application as follows. "There are many, many different challenges and rewards your infant will present you with in the months ahead as you get to know each other. Just as all children change, sometimes dramatically, over weeks and months, [infant's name] will change. Let's look together at what we see him [her] doing right now."

In the authors' experience, the facilitator usually touches the infant more and models more interactions than in the FANA. One mother said, "It was good to see the facilitator hug Mary and call her 'Sweetie' in such an affectionate way. I realized then how lovable Mary could be and that more than anything, she was a baby!"

As with any infant, the whole range of infant competencies and challenges are seen. With the most involved of the infants, one may see very low tone, drooling, a poor suckling reflex, and difficulty in bringing the infant to an alert state.

Tim, the second of two children, had very low tone, difficulty sucking, and had not been able to come to an alert state. During the NBAS application, his mother was able to elicit several reflexes: the babinski, plantar, and palmar grasp. In a light sleep state, Tim turned to his mother's voice and then to his father's voice. His parents were able to see into two windows of their infant's personhood. He could respond when they touched his feet and hands (his mother said she felt as though she had been hugged back) and he showed an interest in his parents' voices—the beginnings of engagement and reciprocal interaction. These first signs of interaction were very reassuring for his mother. It took much longer for his father to feel this way.

There is a small, but growing body of literature on the different responses of mothers and fathers to the birth and rearing of a child with special needs.[11–14] Shonkoff et all[11] reported that fathers of children with Down syndrome had higher parenting stress scores than fathers of children with motor or general developmental delay. Moreover, father of infants with Down syndrome were the only group whose stress was higher than that of the mothers, and fathers' stress was particularly focused on emotional attachment issues. The FANA offers fathers emotional support, concrete assistance, and encouragement to explore the relationship with their newborn.

Not every infant with Down syndrome presents with low tone and is unresponsive. In fact, the more common scenario is an infant with excellent tone, alert to the parental voice, and possessing good state organization. One mother said, "She's just like my other baby." The father remarked, "Big deal! It'll change!" Another father asked, "Does this mean he's normal?" The facilitator cannot give false hope. An appropriate response is, "Development does slow down with infants with Down syndrome, but every infant is different. What we're learning about today is how 'knowable' your newborn is right now and what you need to do to discover as much as you can about each other right now. This exercise will set the stage for years to come."

With one family the FANA was completed again at 2 weeks and at 4 weeks postpartum. Over time it became evident that if the infant was snugly swaddled, and gently bounced 3 to 4 times, she would open her eyes, tighten her facial muscles, make eye contact, and once, she even smiled. It was hard work for the parents to alert her but the payoff was terrific. Her father was ecstatic and said, "I have a game to play with her now." The mother, speaking of her older child, said, "I had no idea how even as a baby he started playing with us. He captured us, but we have to capture her." While the interactional work rested almost exclusively with the parents, they had found a way to begin to interrelate.

Parents speak forcefully about how important it is for them to see their infant respond. For example, one parent explained, "What was so good about the FANA was she was not just sitting there. She was responding! Right at that moment, we felt some relief. That at least she was doing this. She could see me and she could hear me." Parents also comment that they might not have seen these behaviors if left to find them on their own: "With her circumstances, it was just so overwhelming that first week. I just think that we probably would not have noticed much of anything. We were just so upset at that point." Comments such as these reinforce the need for families to have the opportunity to see the infant's behavior in the hospital. One family stated, "It was so good to have seen him interacting. When we got home he was extremely jaundiced, and he slept for the first 4 weeks of his life. I was afraid that he was sleeping because of his Down syndrome, but I remembered what he *had* done in the hospital and that helped me keep the faith."

Parents may also need an opportunity to feel the disappointment created by their infant's responses. "Lisa never gives me a chance to calm her. She doesn't cry . . . she just whimps every 3 hours." This lack of response can be deflating for parents because the neonatal cry leads to parental soothing strategies, which in turn may promote a sense of parental mastery, engagement, and attachment. The task of the facilitator is to confirm the parental observations and acknowledge the sadness and disappointment that can be associated with it.

In the integrative summary, the facilitator provides an opportunity to bring the parents back to their original observations and to reflect on these in light of their infant's behavioral responses. For families with infants with Down syndrome, the summary also offers time to focus on the transition home and on the resources available to families. During this phase, the facilitator has the opportunity to address many questions and provide anticipatory guidance. Some things the facilitator may want to observe are:

- how similar or discordant the parents are in their view of the infant and in their attempts to cope,
- how strong the family's social support network is, and
- what kind of assistance the family needs in order to connect with community resources that are of interest to them.

The facilitator may take time to answer the parents' questions relative to their areas of concern or note the questions and direct them to an appropriate person. At this stage, it is often helpful to focus again on the infant's typicalness.

During the first days, parents may feel that everything about their newborn is unfamiliar. Seeing and reflecting on typical newborn responses opens up the possibility that this infant is also like other infants. One family recalled, "We remembered that our other children were doing these things. It helped us overcome our feelings that everything was going to be different." A first-time father said, "The facilitator was good at picking out strengths. You hear so many negative things in the beginning, a real positive outlook is important. Pick out the good things. Seeing our baby attend and respond was really important because she was inattentive for what seemed like such a long time." Another father's favorite part of the FANA was the facilitator's "loving response to my son, at a time when I didn't know how I felt."

The extent of developmental delay and the nature of the developmental course are as varied with the infant with Down syndrome as they are with any other infant with a disabling condition. While some degree of disability is certain, the characteristics of the environment, the stability of the infant's medical status, and other variables will significantly affect how the infant develops. The facilitator need not be an expert on Down syndrome but must have enough knowledge to reflect and discuss parental questions and to link families with expert consultation. The facilitator must be comfortable handling infants with Down syndrome and must have a general understanding of both the developmental course for infants with Down syndrome and the behavioral subsystems included in the NBAS (ie, habituation, reflexes and tone, orientation, and state regulation). Most important, the facilitator must be able to maintain a receptive and steadying posture that fully accepts the family's emotional responses and that respects and reflects the wholeness and integrity of this new life.

Regardless of the future developmental course, the FANA process focuses on the fact that each infant is unique and that change will occur. Development is not even. A child who is making progress in one area may not make progress in another for a while. Over the years there are many starts and stops for every child. The FANA highlights development as a two-way street: parents teach their infants, and infants teach their parents. The desire to be known serves as a powerful human drive. The FANA provides an entry level experience in mutual discovery between the parents and the child.

• • •

The unexpected delivery of an infant with Down syndrome challenges families to call on adaptive strengths rarely needed in other situations. The presence of Down syndrome clashes radically with what parents thought their infant would look like, be like, and aspire to. Existing expectations will have to be revised or even discarded. This process takes time and energy. While the continuum of adaptation only begins in the hospital, the hospital experience should provide parents with unconditional acceptance of any aspect of their emotional response and should establish how they expect to be accepted by any professional with whom they work.

It is clear that the entire hospital protocol from the moment of birth through the time of discharge needs to be rethought in supporting families of infants with Down syndrome. The solution at the authors' institution was to assemble a multidisciplinary team that, with parental input, specified the roles and supportive acts of each professional who comes in contact with the family during the hospital stay. As a result, the FANA is now nested in a hospitalwide coordinated system of support for families.[15] Based on the literature[16,17] as well as the clinical experiences of a range of hospital-based disciplines such as nursing, social work, pastoral care, and medicine, a systematic protocol for support must be developed. As one father stated, "This is a good hospital, but if you want to be a great hospital, you must address the emotional needs of families." Coming to terms with this request is the challenge for health care systems everywhere.

REFERENCES

1. Cunningham C. *Down's Syndrome: An Introduction for Parents.* Cambridge, Mass: Brookline Books; 1988.
2. Brazelton TB. Family support in the 90s. Presented to Evanston Hospital; May 24, 1990; Evanston, Ill.
3. Wikler L, Wasow M, Hatfield E. Chronic sorrow revisited: Parent vs. professional depiction of the adjustment of parents of mentally retarded children. *Am J Orthopsychiatry.* 1981;51:63–70.
4. Gayton W, Walker L. Down syndrome: Informing the parents. *Am J Dis Child.* 1974;127:510–512.
5. Gath A. Parental reactions to loss and disappointment: The diagnosis of Down syndrome. *Dev Med Child Neurol.* 1985;27:392–400.
6. Shiono H, Kadowaki J-I. The questionnaire to parents of children with Down syndrome: How to inform the parents and psychological responses to counseling. *Am J Med Genet.* 1979;4:215–218.
7. Cardone I, Gilkerson L. Family Administered Neonatal Activities: An innovative component of family centered care. *Zero Three.* 1989;10:23–28.
8. Cardone I, Gilkerson L. Family Administered Neonatal Activities: A first step in the integration of parental perceptions and newborn behavior. *Inf Ment Health J.* 1990;11:127–131.
9. Brazelton TB. *The Neonatal Behavioral Assessment Scale.* Philadelphia, Pa: Lippincott; 1973.
10. Emde R, Brown C. Adaptation to the birth of a Down's syndrome infant. *J Am Acad Child Psychiatry.* 1978;17:299–323.
11. Shonkoff J, Hauser-Cram P, Kraus M, Upshur C. *The Early Intervention Collaborative Study: Final Report of Phase One.* Worcester, Mass: University of Massachusetts Medical School; 1990.

12. Damrosch S, Perry L. Self-reported adjustment, chronic sorrow, and coping of parents and children with Down syndrome. *Nurs Res.* 1989;38:25–30.

13. McLinden S. Mothers' and fathers' reports of the effects of a young child with special needs on the family. *J Early Intervention.* 1990;14:249–259.

14. Salisbury CL. Stressors of parents with young handicapped and non-handicapped children. *J Div Early Child.* 1987;11:154–160.

15. Cardone I, Kraft S, LaPata R, Lawrence P, Salafsky I. *A Hospital-Based, Multidisciplinary Approach to the Unexpected Delivery of an Infant with Down Syndrome.* Evanston, Ill: Evanston Hospital; 1991.

16. Pueschel S, Murphy A. Counseling parents of infants with Down syndrome. *Postgrad Med.* 1975;58:90–95.

17. Newton R, Newton J. Management of Down's syndrome. In: David T, ed. *Recent Advances in Pediatrics.* Edinburgh, Scotland: Livingstone; 1992.

Grandmothers and grandmothers-to-be: Effects on adolescent mothers and adolescent mothering

Judith S. Musick, PhD
Vice Chairman
The Ounce of Prevention Fund
Chicago, Illinois

> And like I told my mother, *I need somebody to love*, just like she needed somebody.
>
> —Gina, a 16-year-old mother

> It's a joy to them. . . . You'll be surprised. You and your mother can be the worst enemies. Then when you have a baby . . . that's the closest time you can get. Since I've been pregnant, me and my mom—well, me and my mom get along better than my mom and sister do.
>
> —Jory, a 16-year-old mother

MANY OF THE SAME developmental and psychologic issues that originally lead adolescent girls to premature parenthood are carried forward to influence how they raise and relate to their children. Perhaps no issues are as powerful in this regard as those connected to the adolescent's relationship with her own mother. During adolescence—a developmental era distinguished by the reemergence and reworking of attachment and separation issues—motherhood may be the arena in which an adolescent's current problems with her mother, as well as her previous problems and deprivations, are played and replayed. Although influenced by a wide range of social, economic, developmental, and psychologic forces, patterns of teenage child*rearing* as well as child*bearing* are powerfully shaped by the mother–daughter relationship, in both its past and present incarnations. Because they are products of the adolescent's adaptations to the realities of her own mother's life as she was growing up, these internal, psychologic models of mothering are not easily changed, especially if they are constantly reinforced by pressures in her current social environment.

Adolescent mothers are a diverse group. Some are extremely capable individuals who require little support or assistance beyond what their family and friends provide; others are less competent, self-destructive, disorganized young women whom no person or intervention seems able to reach or help to any significant

---

Grants from the Rockefeller Foundation and the Harris Foundation enabled me to analyze the data on which this article is based. More recent research carried out under the auspices of the Manpower Demonstration Research Corporation has added greatly to my understanding of multiproblem young mothers and their children. I thank Dr Carol Bryant of the University of South Florida for her generous offer of data from her BEST START breastfeeding study.

Some of the quotes in this article appear in the author's recent book on the psychology of teenage motherhood (see Reference 1). An earlier version of this article was presented in March 1993 at the Conference of the Society for Research in Child Development, New Orleans, Louisiana.

Inf Young Children 1994; 6(3): 1–9

degree. Most, however, fall somewhere between these extremes—performing adequately, or even quite well, as parents, but at some cost to their own development as students or workers. Conversely, some young mothers are able to fulfill their own developmental destiny, but at the cost of that of their child.[1] There are many reasons for this variation in functioning, from personal differences in mental health and basic ability to the amount and quality of family and community support available. For example, some young mothers (and, by extension, their children) thrive because of the consistent, appropriate support they receive from their own mothers and other family members during pregnancy and afterwards. Others pay dearly for whatever support they receive. Still others are compelled, by necessity as well as by duty or guilt, to spend substantial time caring for their younger siblings, or, as is increasingly the case today, to care for a mother with crippling alcohol, drug, or mental health problems of her own. In the isolated, resource-poor social context of poverty today, such reverse-role caretaking takes a heavy toll on the adolescent's own development and, by extension, on that of her child.

Much has been said about the connection between poverty and adolescent childbearing. Yet adolescent parenthood and its sequelae are not simply social and economic problems. They are developmental and psychologic ones as well. This is precisely why they are so complex and difficult to solve. An examination of developmental and psychologic processes is essential for understanding how patterns of teenage pregnancy and parenting are passed from generation to generation. Processes concerned with mother–daughter relations are central to this understanding.

DATA SOURCES AND METHODOLOGY

Much can be learned about the motivations underlying adolescent childrearing behaviors by observing the transactions between young mothers and the interventions designed to help them improve their lives as parents and as people. In that spirit, the ideas presented here are based on studies of participants in programs offering a range of educational, vocational, health, and social services for disadvantaged young women and children. The young women are African-American (40%), white (40%), and Hispanic (Mexican and Puerto Rican) (20%). They live in small towns, rural areas, and large cities in the Midwest and Southeastern regions of the country. Most are single or were so when they first gave birth. All are from poor families, but some are much poorer than others. On the pages that follow, the words of these young mothers, taken from interviews, focus groups, questionnaires, and journals, are used to illustrate the ideas presented. There were six main sources of data:

1. Follow-up interviews with 25 adolescent mothers 18 months after their participation in four urban adolescent parent programs developed by the Ounce of Prevention Fund (OPF), a statewide network of community-

based teen parent programs in Illinois. The study examined former program participants' status in four areas: education, employment, reproductive behavior, and parenting. The data reported here concern the influence of mothers on adolescent daughters' educational, occupational, and personal accomplishments, as well as how mother–daughter relationships were (or were not) affected by program participation.

2. Focus group interviews with 46 pregnant and parenting teens in OPF programs concerning their attitudes about adoption, abortion, and keeping their child. These interviews cover issues of sexuality, feelings about motherhood, and the influence of teens' mothers on their decisions about pregnancy and parenthood.
3. Findings from a survey of 445 pregnant and parenting adolescents in OPF programs on the prevalence of sexual abuse during childhood and adolescence.[2] This was the first study of its kind to examine possible connections between a history of sexual victimization and adolescent childbearing. The data graphically illustrate the coercive nature of sexual and gender socialization for many poor females and highlight the role of the adolescent's own mother in modeling sexual behavior and passivity in relation to males. The data point to confusing messages about sexuality and repeated failures to protect young daughters from men who physically and sexually abuse them.
4. Observations and interviews concerning the causes and correlates of closely spaced, subsequent childbearing among OPF program participants. These data reveal the tendencies of some young mothers to "use" childbearing to avoid the emotional risks of positive change—change that threatens to estrange them from emotionally significant people, especially mothers and other female relatives.
5. Selected material from 35 focus group interviews with economically disadvantaged women in six Southeastern states collected as part of a study of BEST START: Breastfeeding for Healthy Mothers and Healthy Babies (WIC program participants).[3] The study concerns factors influencing young mothers' choices of feeding methods for their infants, but the data are equally pertinent to a range of other issues, including motivation for childbearing, pregnancy resolution choices, and feelings about motherhood; family planning and preventive health care; childrearing practices; attitudes toward marriage; and mother–daughter relations.
6. Diaries and journals of adolescent mothers participating in two programs developed by the Ounce of Prevention Fund: Heart-to-Heart and Dear Diary. Heart-to-Heart was developed in response to repeated disclosures of a history of sexual abuse among pregnant and parenting teens in programs, and on the sexual-abuse prevalence survey mentioned above. Heart-to-Heart aims to prevent sexual abuse by strengthening the abilities of adoles-

cent mothers, especially current or former victims of abuse, to protect their children from sexual as well as other forms of victimization. The centerpiece of Heart-to-Heart is journal writing. Dear Diary incorporates journal writing as part of an ongoing parent support program. The diaries and "journal dialogues" from these two interventions provide critical insights about the internal as well as external forces that shape adolescents' attitudes and actions as parents, partners, and daughters.

Synthesis and interpretation of these sources of evidence yielded information on the role of mother–daughter relations in the teen's desire to be mother—that is, on her motivations for motherhood—and on the caregiving environment she provides once faced with the realities of parenting.

MOTHER–DAUGHTER THEMES

Adolescent pregnancy

Analyses of the various data sets described above revealed a number of prominent developmental themes testifying to the role of grandmothers and grandmothers-to-be in promoting (or preventing) teenaged childbearing, in motivating and enabling their daughters to improve their lives (or to stay where they are), and in shaping their daughters' attitudes and behaviors toward their children. Among these themes are (1) the use of childbearing as compensation for what the teen had failed to get from her mother when she was younger—and the grandmother's direct or indirect support for this motive; (2) the effects of a strongly ambivalent mother–daughter relationship manifested in the girl's rivalry and desire to be better than her mother, balanced by her equally strong fear of being different from her; and (3) the use of childbearing to effect a rapprochement between the girl and her mother during a turbulent time, defusing a potentially explosive situation that threatens emotional separation/loss for both.[1]

The mother–daughter relationship has a distinct and preeminent place in the motivation for a child in one's teens. Because mothers serve such a vital role in their daughters' ego development and individuation efforts,[4] adolescent girls often fear their mothers' power over their lives. As one young woman in Apter's study of mothers and daughters during adolescence describes it, "When I'm angry with my father, I want to punch him; but when I'm angry with my mother, it's as though something's ripping me up inside."[5(p95)] Mother–daughter relations, both negative and positive aspects, are forces to be reckoned with in teenage childbearing, as indicated by the following exchange:

Young mother: I didn't want no children to tell you the truth about it. Every time my mamma would ask, "When you gonna have children?" I

> said, "I ain't planning on having no children," and the next year I was pregnant.
>
> *Interviewer:* How old were you when your mom said that to you?
>
> *Young mother:* I was 16.

Themes testifying to the power of the mother–daughter relationship are woven throughout the various data sets. One finds both childhood themes of previous longing for the mother's love (indeed, even for her presence) and present feelings of love/hostility toward the mother. Such themes testify to the teen's rivalry with her mother, but also demonstrate the teen's dread of the price that she might pay for outshining her. Repeatedly the diaries and interviews tell girls' stories about "telling mama" about the pregnancy; of the anxiety they experienced before telling her; and, significantly, of the enormous relief they felt after having done so. If the girl feels guilty for acting out her rivalry with her mother ("*I* can be a mother too!"), she may be relieved to find that her pregnancy has not permanently estranged her from her mother. If she unconsciously wants a child to validate her mother's lifestyle choices, she may be relieved to find that she has correctly intuited what her mother also wanted, consciously or unconsciously.

Frequently a teen will say that her mother remarked that she had already suspected that her daughter might be pregnant because she had a dream or "sixth sense" about it. The grandmother-to-be may initially be upset, but before too long she and her daughter make up, and the grandmother-to-be begins preparing for the baby to come. This is especially the case for a first grandchild. Such events have extraordinary emotional force in the minds of young mothers. Told and retold as stories, they become part of the personal myth the girl constructs about herself, as a mother and as a daughter. Narratives about telling one's mother, watching and weighing her reaction, also illustrate the ways in which a pregnancy can bring about a rapprochement between a mother at the end of her rope and her rebellious adolescent daughter, defusing a potentially explosive situation. They show us how a pregnancy can allay anxiety for mother and daughter at a point of separation and threatened loss for both, and how it can offer the grandmother-to-be a second chance to do for her grandchild what she was too young or troubled or burdened to do for her daughter when she was a child. Gradually assimilated into the chronicle that the young woman creates about herself as a mother, the story of her mother's response comes to play a part as meaningful as the birth itself.

> My father had me crying and always upset when I first found out I was pregnant. . . . He hurt me so bad I want[ed] to leave home, but my mother she stood by me and still is standing by me. . . . Thank God my mom loves me.

> I was just, like, I was a wall. I didn't know what to do. About a week later everything was OK, cause me and my mom, we was like sisters.
>
> For awhile she didn't speak to me. . . . But she likes it now. She's alright . . . she got me a baby bed for Christmas.
>
> *Question:* What do you think it will it be like when your baby is first born?
>
> *Answer:* My mom holding it all the time. [Her tone is almost cooing with love.]
>
> I was having an abortion and my mom said no, cause this is her first grandchild. I believe that's why she wanted it. She's excited about it.
>
> My mother, she was sitting in the room, so she said, "You are pregnant," like that. So my mamma, she looked at me, and I felt her looking, but I didn't look back at her. She just said, "Well ya'll have a baby to take care of." But I feel like she was happy because by the next month she was going buying the baby this, getting the baby that.

Mother–daughter relations are highly complex, as complex as the individuals themselves. Grandmothers often suffer from an abundance of unmet needs themselves. If they lack alternative means of gratification, they may look to their children as potential sources rather than recipients of nurturance. Thus they sometimes use them to fulfill their unmet needs.[6] A grandmother may not welcome her daughter's pregnancy, especially if she is still quite young and in her own childbearing and childrearing years. Still, many women, especially poor women, are fatalistic in outlook, feeling that the matter is out of their control.

> [My mom] fussed for awhile and finally, when she accepted it, it was alright between us. . . . It's too late to be mad now. They accepted it now.
>
> No, they wasn't mad. It's over with now. Ain't nothing to be done. That's why my mamma didn't fuss.

It also seems likely that a mother might feel a need to make up for her past failures by reworking unresolved parenting issues with a new generation. Regretting her inability to devote sufficient time or emotional energy to her own children when they were younger, she may seek to give to a grandchild what she was too busy, encumbered, or immature to give to the child's mother. In this way the grandmother can make amends for earlier deprivations, expressing her love for her daughter through her love of the child she has produced, redoing and (she hopes) undoing the past.

The nature of a girl's relationship to her mother, past and present, plays a significant part in determining how successfully she meets and masters the developmental challenges of adolescence. It is harder, for example, to resolve adolescent issues of separation and individuation if the childhood mother–daughter relationship was unsatisfactory. Even under "normal" conditions, the physical and psychologic changes brought about by adolescence tend to reawaken strong wishes to be nurtured by and to be close to a mothering figure. (Anna Freud[7] viewed these essentially normal regressions as being in the service of ego development, that is, they are especially useful in helping the young person to meet and manage developmental challenges.) Regressions of this kind can make the normal challenges of the adolescent transitional period seem formidable, if not insurmountable, if there is a history of troubled mother–daughter relations. In such cases early fertility can be viewed as one way for the adolescent girl to meet her need to be psychologically connected to her mother, to recapitulate her experiences, and to gain some badly needed comfort and emotional sustenance from her. It is not at all unusual for a pregnant teenager to discuss such longings quite openly, articulating her hope that her "plight" will result in a maternal change of heart, eliciting the loving care of which she feels deprived. Quite often it does. The grandmother-to-be may initially act angry or distraught, but eventually she comes around. The psychic rewards will be forthcoming, at least for a while.

Such themes have been observed in previous studies. For example, clinical observations of teen parents[8] indicate that pregnancy often creates a moratorium, bringing a rebellious young woman closer to her mother and allowing her a means of separating in a more modulated way. It affords her the opportunity to assert her autonomy without sacrificing intimacy, especially if she knows or intuits that her mother would like a grandchild. The impending birth of a child may help to resolve the painful struggles around separation and dependency that are experienced by many teens, struggles that are even more highly charged in conflict-laden mother–daughter relationships, where there is a history of attachment problems or where a mother has been present only intermittently or sporadically for much of her daughter's life.

Adolescent parenting

Some adolescents actually do straighten out as their pregnancy advances or after the birth of the child. Motherhood seems to serve as a psychologic catalyst for these adolescents, a way to stop them from really destroying their lives. For many it is a sort of self-administered "ah ha!" experience or a psychologic wake-up call. (Osofsky, Osofsky, and Diamond[9] present an interesting description of how the transition to parenthood is negotiated by adolescent mothers.)

> This baby's wising me up to know I gotta get out there and make it for myself.

> . . . I got pregnant . . . and that's when I settled down. . . . That's how I straightened myself out, by getting pregnant.

Considering the significance of the mother–daughter relationship during the early and middle adolescent years, it is possible that this phenomenon is at least partly a consequence of the twin comforts experienced by the girl in effecting a rapprochement with her mother and in avoiding an emotionally tumultuous and precipitous separation for which she is developmentally and psychologically unprepared. For some girls the central task of adolescence—moving toward adulthood—can be accomplished by identifying with the mother and her way of life, a separation without psychologic amputation. The young woman now views herself (and knows that others view her) as a changed, more adult-like person. Yet at the same time she remains a vital limb on her family's tree.

Parenting requires the adolescent to take on a new set of duties that call for distinctive skills and higher levels of maturity. If she is successful in accomplishing these duties (and if others, such as the grandmother, have not completely taken over the care of the child) she gains a new and highly rewarding sense of proficiency, a sense of personal worth she may never have experienced before. The satisfactory resolution of developmental and psychologic issues through the bearing and caring for children does indeed free some young women from a kind of self-limiting psychologic imprisonment. It enables them to move ahead and succeed in other areas and roles such as school or work. There is a catch, however. Those adolescents who manage to put motherhood to good developmental use almost always have substantial support from others and substantial personal and social resources themselves. While such adolescents may "rise to the occasion" of motherhood, others, devoid of these resources, plunge to the depths, pulling their children along with them.

Balancing child development with personal development calls for maturity, psychologic strength, and a full complement of family and outside supports. To be a student and/or an employee, a daughter, friend, partner, and a mother is demanding under any circumstances. To do so at the age of 16 or 17 years, in a milieu where there is absolutely no margin for error, calls for extraordinary skills and strengths. Without such skills and strengths, someone unavoidably will be short changed. All too often that someone will be the adolescent's child. Quite often this will be due to her relations with men, stemming from the legacy of her history as witness and, perhaps, even casualty of her own mother's relationships with men and of the messages these relationships imparted about motherhood.

> Like maybe you didn't have your mother's and father's love when you were growing up, so you always depend on the opposite sex—as long as they tell you they love you, you put them before anything. You will put them before your kids . . . and why? I mean, you're not talking about

> marriage; it is just going to be a fling. The kids are there, supposed to be there, for life.

The nature of the relationships of the girl's mother with men and, equally relevant, of the girl's place in such relationships when she was growing up can have enduring—and deadly—effects on her later capacity for raising and relating to her own children. Consider the following statements:

> We didn't understand until we got our nerve to tell my mom what he was doing. But when we did, she didn't believe us. . . . I even thought it was a dream since she didn't believe us and he was still in her life . . . and my mom had a baby from him. [This teenage mother and her sister were repeatedly abused by their mother's boyfriend.]

> Mothers should be real careful about the people they date or people they plan to get married with . . . and don't ever choose a man over your own flesh and blood.

> I had a sexual experience with my mother's boyfriend. He made me suck on his penis and he made me kiss him. I was 12 years old.

Adolescent mothers such as these frequently end up repeating a pattern whereby a child is sacrificed to maintain a relationship with a man (or, over a period of years, a number of men) on whom the woman is emotionally dependent.

> It really bothers me to see [my daughters] go through the same thing I did when I was younger. I was sexually abused when I was 7 until 11½ years. I tried to forget it, but when it happened to my little girl, it all came back again.

> I have a lot of girlfriends who go through the same problem too, and they're in the same situation as me. . . . They're just in a messed-up apartment with their kids, and their boyfriends are druggies or gang bangers and . . . the guys are putting their lives in danger, not only theirs but their kids . . . and they don't really care.

Relationships with men

Tragically, the lives of many teenage (and former teenage) mothers are ruled by the need to get and keep a man. Repeatedly seeking and involving themselves in self-destructive relationships with males, these psychologically vulnerable teens are victimized time after time.

> I feel like a big piece of *gum,* the kind that sticks to a shoe and gets stepped on, over and over again. I've tried everything to keep him.

The children of victims are frequently victims themselves, the heirs of their mothers' entanglements in unstable, abusive relationships. In her struggle for emotional survival, an adolescent mother may sacrifice her child to her need for emotional support from a man. The stresses and costs of such "support" are borne by children as much as, possibly even more than, their mothers.

> He's not normal I guess. . . . He sometimes is rough with the kids. Two weeks ago he slapped Claudia across her face. He did this around 1 in the afternoon. When I came home from school I noticed the marks. . . . She had broken veins on her face. . . . I hate Matt because he is mean. . . . If I do a lot of things and play with the kids a lot, Matt says I'm ignoring him. He's jealous. A family isn't supposed to be like that. I don't know what's wrong with our family that makes it like it is. What can I do?

Physical or sexual abuse, neglect, even abandonment are only the most obvious and readily apparent consequences of young mothers' enmeshments with domineering or dangerous men. But the psychologic pressure, indeed the compulsion, to please a man—to gain and retain his support—may take a myriad of forms, touching virtually any parenting function and compromising the quality of the relationship itself.

> Dear Lindsey, Today Mommy felt really bad about Rusty [the mother's much older boyfriend] treating me wrong, and I didn't feel like hearing you cry. But you know that I really love you and care about you.

> My fiancee don't want me to breast-feed. . . . He don't think that these belong to the baby, they belong to him. . . . He thinks they're for a sexual thing [more] than it is as far as a health thing.

Thus when a teenage mother is overdependent on her relationships with men, new risk is added to an already risk-laden environment. This, in turn, deprives those children in greatest jeopardy of precisely those benefits most likely to prevent, reduce, or remediate developmental damage.

DISCUSSION

The diaries, interviews, and focus group discussions give a vivid picture of the special meanings that children hold for young mothers, some of which are distinct from those shared with mothers who are older. It is these separate meanings—as much as adolescent immaturity per se, or lack of knowledge of child development, or difficult life circumstances per se, or child characteristics—that determine what a teen actually does as a mother. As can be seen, the children of adolescents are more likely to be encumbered by their mothers' past and current relationship problems with their mothers and with their expectation that the rewards of parenthood—rewards that make up for past deprivations—should come from what children give to parents, not the reverse. The adolescent's child is also more likely to be burdened by his young mother's unrealistic dreams and hopes, that is, unconsciously blamed and treated harshly (possibly rejected) for failing to solve her developmental problems or for not providing the "cure" for her sadness or self-doubt. Still so young, so full of unfulfilled maternal longings, how can she give her child what she so badly needs herself? How can she actively and proactively foster her child's development within the mother–child relationship when she is still so caught up with her own? Not fully developed, an adolescent mother may not yet be capable of a truly reciprocal parenting relationship. She may be too self-absorbed to permit, let alone enable, her children to be themselves, free from her needs and projections. Interestingly, what may look like the teen's neglect or pathologic distance from her child may actually be a manifestation of her symbiosis, or lack of differentiation—her inability to distinguish her child's needs from her own.

Day care provider: Did you feed him breakfast this morning?

Adolescent mother: I wasn't hungry.

And, she may not put on his sweater when she is not cold.

IMPLICATIONS FOR INTERVENTION

It is a bitter truth that some young mothers inexorably shape their children's lives into mirror images of their own, not necessarily by design, but by default. This is especially the case if the early mother–daughter relationship was, and has remained, painful and depriving, and if no compensatory experiences with caring others were available to the girl as she grew up. Without such ameliorative experiences, cycles of maternal pathology are likely to pass from generation to generation unbroken. For the children of such young mothers, the best our society can do is to provide high-quality developmental child-care settings where these children can spend a significant part of each day. Realistically, early intervention for these children is more important, and more likely to be successful, than is relatively later intervention aimed at their mothers.

On the other hand, many adolescent mothers with initial parenting problems do establish very good relationships with their children, perhaps not immediately, but eventually. It should be noted, however, that for this to happen, they may need more support and assistance than the average teen parent program alone is likely to provide. They frequently require more intensive, therapeutically or developmentally informed services for themselves and for their children. In addition, they also need at least some of the following: (1) stable living arrangements, since they commonly move around a great deal; (2) better child care, since they often leave their children with a variety of not-so-desirable caretakers; (3) the encouragement (or at least the absence of active discouragement) of a competent, caring male partner; and (4) the support and help of stable, adult family members. Under these circumstances, and with some counseling or therapeutic services, parenting difficulties can be greatly reduced, or even turned around, especially if the young mother makes a deliberate decision to raise her child differently—and better—than she was raised herself,

> I don't want [my children] to say when they get bigger, "my mom beat me up." Now *my* mother threw anything she seen or anything she put her hand on. . . . You're standing there and she hits you with one of these [fist]. I try not to be like that with my kids. . . . I don't want them ever to leave me. Cause I done that to my mother a lot of times.

to recognize that she needs help,

> I thought I knew everything and anything there was to know about being a mother . . . and you just don't know. It is a very hard job which I have to do. . . . I used to feel that I am the only one having a hard time coping with my kids, but I'm glad to know that I'm not. And that there are others . . . and there is help.

and to be willing to make use of the resources available to help her change,

> If it wasn't for this program, I would have raised her just like I was raised.

REFERENCES

1. Musick J. *Young, Poor, and Pregnant: The Psychology of Teenage Motherhood.* New Haven, Conn: Yale University Press; 1993.
2. Gershenson H, Musick J, Ruch-Ross H, Magee V, Rubino K, Rosenberg D. The prevalence of coercive sexual experience among teenage mothers. *J Interpers Violence.* 1989;4(2):204–219.
3. Bryant C, Bailey D, Coreil J, D'Angelo S, Lazarov M. Determinants of Breastfeeding in the Southeast Region: Research Findings from the BEST START: Breastfeeding for Healthy Mothers and Healthy Babies Campaign. Tampa, Fla: University of South Florida, School of Public Health; 1989.
4. Powers S, Hauser S, Schwartz J, Noam G, Jacobson A. Adolescent ego development and family interaction: a structural-developmental perspective. In: Grotevant H, Cooper C, eds. *New Directions for Child Development (Number 22): Adolescent Development in the Family.* San Francisco, Calif: Jossey-Bass; 1983.

5. Apter T. *Altered Loves: Mothers and Daughters During Adolescence.* New York, NY: St. Martin's Press; 1990.
6. Ladner J, Gourdine R. Intergenerational teenage motherhood: some preliminary findings. *SAGE: A Scholarly Journal on Black Women.* 1984;1(2):22–24.
7. Freud A. Instinctual anxiety during puberty. In: *The Writings of Anna Freud: Vol. 2. The Ego and the Mechanisms of Defense.* 2nd ed. New York, NY: International Universities Press; 1966.
8. O'Leary K, Shore M, Weider S. Contacting pregnant adolescents: are we missing cues? *Social Casework.* 1984;65(5):297–306.
9. Osofsky J, Osofsky H, Diamond M. The transition to parenthood: special tasks and risk factors for adolescent parents. In: Michaels G, Goldberg W, eds. *The Transition to Parenthood: Current Theory and Research.* Cambridge, England: Cambridge University Press; 1988.

Dyad as focus, triad as means: A family-centered approach to supporting parent–child interactions

Jeanette A. McCollum, PhD
Professor
Department of Special Education

T. J. Yates, PhD
Coordinator, Partnership Project
Institute for Research on Human Development
University of Illinois
Champaign, Illinois

FAMILY PARTICIPATION is a key tenet of the early intervention movement, guiding the growth of both policy and practice with regard to services for young children (birth to age 3) and their families. As noted almost two decades ago,[1] offering parents a less than integral role in intervention events that affect their children makes little sense from a developmental perspective. This belief has been so strong that a series of articles to the contrary,[2] summarizing results of existing data from multiple programs serving children with disabilities, birth to age 5, was greeted with skepticism and outright controversy.[3,4] A later analysis of data, prompted by the outcry, from programs serving children younger than 3 years yielded very different outcomes; contrary to making no difference, the extent and type of parent involvement emerged as a strong predictor of child outcome.[5] More importantly, however, later research has shown that the influences that families have on their children, and likewise the influences that early intervention programs have on families, are multifaceted and complex. Far more sophistication is emerging in matching what programs expect from and provide to families, with each family's individual concerns and priorities. For instance, it no longer is expected that mothers and fathers have the same concerns or profit from the same types of program opportunities.[6] In addition, greater sophistication is emerging in the measures used to determine whether and how intervention influences families and their children.[7] What has long made developmental sense is increasingly supported by new efficacy research.[8] Furthermore, since the passage in 1986 of Public Law 99-457, it is supported by federal law and policy.

As family policy is translated into practice, it seems critical to understand just what it is about the roles of families in the intervention process that might explain their influence on important child outcomes. Guralnick's[9] review of the "second generation" of efficacy research provides just such a clue: the one factor best differentiating the more successful intervention efforts was the extent to which the interventions were aimed at supporting and enhancing the roles of families as competent and confident caregivers of their young children. Families, not intervention programs, provide continuity in their child's life. They are, by definition, the primary physical and social setting in which the child's development occurs.[10] It is within the emotionally rich family context that children develop the sense of

Inf Young Children 1994; 6(4): 54–63

self and others that colors how they will approach both current and future interactions with their social and physical worlds.[11–13] The view that the parent–child relationship is at the heart of the intervention process is entirely compatible with the philosophy underlying Part H. That philosophy supports practices of early intervention that facilitate and expand the competence and independence in family members with regard to this relationship.

Traditional practices of multiple disciplines have come under increasing scrutiny with regard to their congruence with a family-centered philosophy. This has resulted in broad changes in the roles that families play in state, local, and individual program policy making. It also has led to new guidelines for practice in a number of specific programmatic components, including assessment,[14] Individualized Family Service Plan (IFSP) development,[15–17] and service coordination.[18,19]

One critical aspect of early intervention practice that has received much less scrutiny is the intervention process itself: What is it that professionals do in their interactions with families, and how do they do it? What kinds of relationships, what kinds of interactions and styles of communication during the intervention process, meet the criterion of "family-centeredness"? The answers to these questions seem particularly important if one buys into the central role of the parent, and of the parent–child relationship, in child development.

THE INTERVENTION TRIAD AS AN INTERACTION UNIT

Within our own project, this gap in knowledge became obvious as we began to plan a series of parent–infant play groups that had the following goals:

- to support and expand parent–child interactions that were both pleasurable and developmentally and individually appropriate to each child's level of understanding, physical abilities, and state;
- to establish interventionist–parent interactions that respect and honor the parent;
- to strengthen the parent's sense of competence through guided parent–child interactions that enhance the parent's self-efficacy as a parent;
- to build parenting knowledge and skills that parents could apply beyond the context of the play groups;
- to facilitate parents' recognition of the importance of their own roles in the child's development; and
- to assist parents to take a problem-solving or "hypothesis-setting" orientation to establishing developmentally supportive interactions.

Given these goals, the question for us became: "How?" How do we organize the groups, and, particularly, how do we organize our own interactions with parents within those groups to accomplish these goals? Based on our experience in the initial stages of implementation, a related question became: "How can we accomplish our goals within the context of a group setting in which diversity is the rule, rather than the exception?" We knew that each parent came to the sessions for different reasons. Furthermore, they had different backgrounds, different relationships with their children, and different understandings of their child's development and of their own roles in it, as well as different abilities and learning styles.[20–22]

What emerged from this process was a triadic model that gives explicit attention to the interactions among the three members of the intervention triad: child, parent, and interventionist. The triadic model recognizes the importance of the parent–child interaction by making it a primary focus of the intervention process.[23,24] The goal of the model is to build on and expand the strengths of the parent–infant dyad by providing contextual and interpersonal support for their interactions. The model was designed to give interventionists from multiple disciplines a framework for thinking about typical visits in which they work together with a parent and child (eg, parent–child play group, home visit, in-center therapy session). The triadic strategies to be described in this article directly address the component of the triadic model related to interpersonal interactions among participants, particularly those strategies used by the interventionist to support interactions between parent and child.

The following section describes the triadic strategies, as well as guidelines for their use. Subsequent to this description, the theoretical framework that undergirds the triadic model as a whole will be reviewed briefly.

THE TRIADIC STRATEGIES

The triadic strategies build on the principles of good communication: listening and observing, interpreting, hypothesizing, responding, and evaluating.[25] As shown in the box, "Overview of Triadic Strategies," the six strategies are behaviors already very familiar to most early interventionists. Within the triadic model, however, these behaviors are specifically thought of as strategies to be employed, through the vehicle of the parent–child–interventionist triad,[24] to expand parents' awareness of their childrens' abilities and intents and of their own strengths in supporting these characteristics. It is the conscious awareness and employment of the strategies according to particular guidelines that define their usefulness as "strategies" that will bring the interactions between and among these three primary participants in the intervention process into congruence with the goals stated earlier.

Beginning with the first strategy, the interventionist establishes a supportive context by arranging the environment in a way that increases the probability that playful interactions will occur. This could be accomplished by providing dyadic activities, such as a social game, that encourage the parent and child to face each other and give each partner a role in the interaction. During the course of the inter-

Overview of Triadic Strategies

1. *Establish a supportive context.* Elements of the environment are arranged or rearranged by the interventionist to increase the probability of playful interaction.
2. *Acknowledge parent competence.* Developmentally facilitative behaviors of the parent are warmly recognized and expanded, as are characteristics of child competence.
3. *Focus attention.* Aspects of the interaction are commented on, questioned, or expanded in order to draw the parent's attention to particular competencies or actions.
4. *Provide information.* Information about the child's developmental agenda is given within the context of play.
5. *Model.* Dyadic interaction roles are momentarily taken on by the interventionist.
6. *Suggest.* The parent is given a specific suggestion as to what to do with the child.

action, the interventionist might move slightly to the side of the child, thereby enabling the child to focus attention on the parent. A supportive context undergirds all of the other strategies; many times it may be all that is needed to achieve a developmentally facilitative interaction.

The interventionist using the second strategy unobtrusively acknowledges parental competence by warmly recognizing and expanding on the parent's use of developmentally facilitative behaviors with the child. For example, if the parent is singing a song with the child and the child expresses joy with the interaction, the interventionist might point out to the parent how much the child enjoys the situation and comment on the ways in which this activity supports the child's development. The interventionist may elect to use the same strategy by speaking for the child: "Daddy, I love singing this song together. And you're helping me learn new sounds, too!"

The third strategy focuses the parent's attention on the child by commenting or expanding on particular competencies or actions. For example, if, in the context of a parent–infant play group, the parent often ignores the child to socialize with other parents, the interventionist might direct the parent's attention to the child by commenting on the child's competence ("Look! Katie is trying to open the door with a key!"), or by soliciting related parental input ("Has she ever done that before?").

Within the context of the same play session, the interventionist may use the fourth strategy to provide information about the child's developmental agenda. Thus, in the previous example, after getting the mother to focus on her child's actions, the interventionist might use the opportunity to verbally interpret the developmental issue that the child is working on as she tries to unlock the door with the key.

In the fifth strategy, modeling, the interventionist momentarily takes on the parent's dyadic interaction role. For example, the interventionist might model the parent role in a turn-taking routine, or might act out the parent's role by rolling a ball toward the child and saying, "Let's play. You take a turn and then I'll take a turn." Momentary modeling clarifies alternatives that parents can learn and incorporate into their repertoire of skills; a new context thereby becomes available for supporting parental competence.

The last of the triadic strategies is to give the parent a specific suggestion as to what to do with the child. The interventionist might say to the parent, "Maybe Johnny would like for you to roll the ball to him. What do you think will happen if you do?" He or she might also make a suggestion by talking for the child: "Mommy, let's roll the ball to each other."

The triadic strategies are applied according to a set of guidelines that support their use as a tool in achieving a family-centered interaction. The first guideline is that the specific strategy used at any given moment *must match the individual strengths of the parent.* This is achieved by thinking of these six strategies as constituting a continuum that is defined by the amount of support the interventionist provides to promote the interaction. Thus, in the box, the most open-ended, indirect strategies are at the top, and those providing the most direct support to the interaction are at the bottom. The second guideline is that the interventionist first determines where to start on this continuum and then *follows the parent's lead.* Movement up and down this continuum is determined by the ongoing flow of the interaction. A third guideline is that the interventionist makes continuing judgments about whether the particular strategy selected will be more supportive if it is used with the parent *directly* or *indirectly through taking the child's voice.*[26] The entire process is carried out within a framework of enlisting the parent in *observing and hypothesizing* about what the child is experiencing. Hence, each strategy is designed to be used in a "conversational," natural format and to be imbedded within the context of everyday play and caregiving routines.

In the process of triadic interaction, the interventionist engages in an undergirding process of observation, hypothesizing, responding, and evaluating; judgments are made from moment to moment. The interventionist's efforts are directed toward achieving a balance between providing sufficient support to attain the primary goals (eg, enhancing the parent's self-efficacy as a parent, providing a pleasurable, developmentally supportive context), while simultaneously leaving the parent in charge of the flow of the interaction by following the parent's lead.[17] This is in contrast to more traditional approaches to fostering interactions by relying primarily on more directive modes such as telling parents what to do.[27]

The following example illustrates the use of these strategies and the movement along the continuum from moment to moment within a particular interaction. The interventionist begins by *establishing a supportive environment*: planning a dyadic rattle activity for an adolescent mother and her infant. The mother shakes the brightly colored rattle at her infant, who is on a blanket across the room. To assist the mother to *focus her attention* and reflect on what is happening with her infant, the interventionist asks the parent what she thinks might happen if she held the rattle a little closer to the infant. Mom replies, "I don't know" and makes no attempt to move closer to the infant. The interventionist then *suggests* to the mother that she move closer to the infant, gently shake the rattle, and observe what her infant does. The mother is hesitant. The interventionist then momentarily *models*, gently shaking the rattle closer to the baby, at the same time *providing information* by interpreting how the infant is showing that she likes the rattle (eg, smiling, kicking her feet, and reaching). Mother then tries the activity, and the interventionist *acknowledges the parent's competence* by commenting on the child's positive response to the mother's actions. Within this interaction, all six triadic strategies were employed. At each step the interventionist observed the parent's response, made a judgment about which strategy to use next, and then reevaluated again, providing more or less support in response to the mother's participation.

The interventionist who integrates these strategies into ongoing interactions with parents is using the interventionist–parent relationship to model a parallel relationship between parent and child[17]—one based on reading cues, hypothesizing, and responding. Good observation skills and a sound knowledge of child development are central to using the triadic strategies continuum.

THE TRIADIC MODEL'S FIT WITH THEORY

The theoretical framework that undergirds the triadic model is derived from four somewhat disparate bodies of literature. One area that contributed heavily to the development of the model is the literature on parent–infant interaction. This literature indicates that interactions with persons with whom the child has strong emotional ties have important implications not only for the continuity and health of that particular relationship,[28] but also for the predispositions that the child brings to future interactions and relationships with other persons.[29,30] The development of a sense of self-efficacy, mastery, and competence with regard to expectations that one can control one's environment[31] are influenced by parent–infant interactions that support the child's emerging emotional sense of self. Thus, the feedback that an infant receives from emotionally salient individuals early in life appear to be critically important to development. Alternatively, parents' sense of self-efficacy as parents are dependent on the responses of the infant to their efforts in play and caregiving.[31,32]

Underlying those interactions that are satisfying to both partners are qualities such as responsiveness and matching.[33] However, when one partner is an infant, the burden of carrying the interaction rests with the infant's partner. The ability of the adult partner to read the infant's state and intent and to adjust his or her own interactions accordingly are critical to the emotions that both partners will experience about themselves and one another. In cases in which the infant has a disability or other biologic difference that may interfere with readability,[32,34] the "readerability" necessary on the parent's part may be even greater, and yet more difficult.[27] Individual differences among parents in the ability to read their infants' cues also may interfere with this interactive match.[13,20]

The parent–child interaction literature as a whole indicates that these interactions should be an integral part of the early intervention process. The triadic model is designed to directly facilitate characteristics of interaction that support the child's optimal development.

Infant mental health, with its emphasis on relationships, is a second body of literature that has guided development of the triadic model. This literature emphasizes the centrality of early relationships with caregivers in the child's development, reinforcing the importance of explicitly recognizing the importance of these relationships within the intervention process. Expanding beyond the parent–child interaction literature, it draws attention to the importance of taking into account the "lenses" through which parents see their children.[26,35] That is, the parent's perception of the interaction will be based not only on what is occurring within any particular situation or what has occurred in similar situations in the past, but also on the values and beliefs that the parent has about children in general and about this child in particular. These values and beliefs may be broadly based in the culture[36] or strictly individual, reflecting that individual's own early experience of family and parenting.[37]

For the interventionist working with the parent–child dyad, this implies the need to listen and observe, to make hypotheses, and to check them out with the parent through discussion. It also implies that the interventionist must recognize and evaluate the influence that his or her own values and beliefs may have on interpersonal interactions with this dyad.[38] Thus, in essence, the interventionist–parent relationship will be most powerful when it mirrors the qualities of the parent–child relationship and is in keeping with the intervention goals.[39] An important role of the interventionist is to assist the parent in "knowing" the child by modeling strategies for knowing and respecting the parent.[40,41] "Do unto others as you would have them do unto others" is an important theme of the triadic model (E. Fenichel, personal communication, 1992).

Literature on empowerment and enablement, which undergirds the family-centered movement as a whole,[42] also contributed to the development of the triadic model. The concept of empowerment implies that, for intervention to have lasting effects, the individual must perceive that changes or outcomes are due to his or her own efforts, rather than to the efforts of another person. Enablement implies that, to achieve this, individuals must have access to the information and skills necessary to achieve success and must be able to link these resources to their own efforts. The family-centered guidelines emerging from these concepts emphasize a proactive approach that builds on and expands families' own resources and strengths.[42] This is accomplished by ensuring that families' choices within the intervention process are respected and followed, as well as by giving explicit recognition to the strengths that families bring to parenting and to intervention. This process is enhanced by providing access to the information and skills that family members may need in order to make informed choices about their child's program and about their own roles.

These principles are interwoven throughout the triadic interaction model. The structural component of the model is designed to set up conditions that leave maximum control of the intervention situation with the parent. This theme is carried over into the triadic strategies, which leave the parent in charge of the parent–child interaction so that the child's success will be a result of the parent's own efforts (empowerment), while at the same time using the interaction situation to provide developmental information that may assist the parent in achieving more pleasurable and developmentally supportive interactions (enablement). Underlying the careful balance between these two principles is ongoing, thoughtful interpretation of and responsiveness to the parent's perspective.

The fourth literature that has contributed substantially to the triadic model is that on the zone of proximal development, particularly that portion of the literature related to scaffolding.[43] Although developed primarily within the context of cognitive and language learning, the concept of scaffolding provides a very useful framework for interactions with adults as well. Scaffolding refers to the type and amount of support provided by the individual with more information, during the process of assisting the second individual to achieve the same knowledge. The role of the scaffolder is to offer enough assistance to enable the learner to perform slightly beyond his or her current level, and thereby to grow, without providing too much assistance or taking control of the situation away from the learner. Scaffolding also is based on the premise that the scaffolder must be able to modify the degree and type of support, not only across persons, based on the abilities that they bring to the situation, but also with the same individual across contexts.[44] Modifications also must occur on a moment-by-moment basis within the particular situation as the learner achieves new levels of competence and encounters new problems to be solved.

The usefulness of the concept of scaffolding to the triadic model lies first in its emphasis on the balance between the amount and type of support needed and desired by the individual learner, and that provided by the scaffolder. In addition, the model emphasizes that the learner is acquiring not just skills, but generalizable principles that will make sense and be usable in many similar situations. Finally, the learner is placed in an active role, with the motivation for learning stemming from his or her own efforts within an emotionally important situation; therefore, what is gained from the scaffolder makes sense within the context in which the learner is currently engaged. Within the triadic model, the interventionist acts as a scaffolder for the parent–child dyad, as well as fostering the parent's ability to scaffold interactions with the child.

Concepts derived from these four bodies of literature have provided the framework that underlies the triadic model. Taken together, they indicate that the role of the interventionist is indeed complex, requiring a unique blend of self-knowledge and readerability, in-depth knowledge of child development, and extraordinary interpersonal skills. Equally as important, however, these literatures point to the significance of how interventions are carried out. The basic premise of the triadic model is that interventions will be most powerful if the "how" is explicitly chosen to be congruent with the "what."[27] This is reflected in the parallel processes occurring between parent and child and between interventionist and parent. The roles of the interventionist, and the strategies used in interaction with the parent, therefore assume primary importance.[45]

SUMMARY AND DISCUSSION

A family-centered perspective demands that those in the early intervention field review and scrutinize practice for its compatibility not only with new policy, but also with the philosophy and values that undergird this perspective.[27] The triadic interaction model was specifically designed to reflect these standards, drawing its framework from four disparate but compatible bodies of literature. Although the model was developed within the context of early intervention directed explicitly toward the parent–child dyad, we believe that the model applies equally to situations in which the parent–child interaction provides the context and vehicle for more child-focused intervention (eg, physical therapy) or in which the intervention is more parent focused (eg, social work).[46] It also appears to be applicable across the different types of settings (eg, home visits, play groups) in which parent, child, and interventionist participate.

Despite this apparent compatibility, we acknowledge the potential limitations of this model. For instance, basic needs such as housing may momentarily preempt the family's ability to focus emotional attention on their relationship with their infant. Other parents may come with emotional needs of their own that cannot be addressed through the parent–infant interaction, but rather must be addressed separately and perhaps first. All families come with their own configurations of cultural and personal values, each having implications for their views of the parent–child relationship, of professional roles, and of appropriate communication between themselves and interventionists.[47] These may influence the applicability of some or all of the components of the triadic interaction process. However, the premises of the model appear to accommodate these as well. Family-centeredness is not a set of particular practices, but rather an attitude and a way of thinking about families in which families are recognized as having unique concerns, strengths, and values; as a result, family-centered interaction may be very different for each family. One of the central premises of the triadic model is that what the interventionist provides must match what the parent perceives as being important within the context of the interaction. Therefore, not employing particular strategies is a viable option within this model.

Although the triadic strategies presented in this article are relatively straightforward and concrete, the ability of any individual interventionist to employ them will be influenced by a complex combination of personal and situational factors. Adopting a triadic model has important implications, not only for program policy and practice, but also for training and for the supervisory process. Interventionists using this model must have an excellent working knowledge of child development, be able to think on their feet, monitor multiple interactions occurring from moment to moment, and have the capacity to alter their own behavior in response to what they observe. Within a preservice setting, students will need opportunities to assume and practice these roles, supported by a supervisor who mirrors these same processes in interactions with the student.[48] Similarly, at the inservice level, interventionists will need the support of supervisors who provide the same kinds of interactive opportunities.[49] Because each individual enters the intervention situation with his or her own history and values, both preservice and inservice settings must focus on assisting each interventionist to examine his or her own perspectives and to recognize how these perspectives color his or her relationships with families and children.

The parent–infant dyad is, by definition, a critical unit within the early intervention system. Recognition of this unit clearly is an important component of the intervention process. The triadic strategies described in this article were designed to support and strengthen the dyadic relationship through recognizing and building on the importance of the self-efficacy and competence of the parent in the parenting role.

REFERENCES

1. Bronfenbrenner U. Is early intervention effective? In: Frielander B, Sterritt G, Kirk G, eds. *Exceptional Infant: Assessment and Intervention.* New York, NY: Brunner/Mazel;1975.
2. Casto G, Mastropieri M. The efficacy of early intervention programs: a metaanalysis. *Except Child.* 1986;53:417–424.
3. Dunst C, Snyder SW. A critique of the Utah State University early intervention meta-analysis research. *Except Child.* 1985;52:269–276.
4. Strain PS, Smith GJ. A counter-interpretation of early intervention effects: a response to Casto and Mastropieri. *Except Child.* 1986;53:260–265.
5. Shonkoff J, Hauser-Cram P. Early intervention for disabled infants and their families: a quantitative analysis. *Pediatrics.* 1987;80:650–658.

6. Upshur C. Mothers' and fathers' ratings of the benefits of early intervention services. *J Early Intervention.* 1992;15:345–357.
7. Guralnick MJ. The next decade of research on the effectiveness of early intervention. *Except Child.* 1991;58:174–183.
8. Shonkoff JP, Hauser-Cram P, Krauss MW, Upshur CC. Development of infants with disabilities and their families. *Monogr Soc Res Child Dev.* 1992;57(serial no. 230).
9. Guralnick MJ. Recent developments in early intervention efficacy research: implications for family involvement in P.L. 99-457. *Top Early Child Spec Educ.* 1989;9:1–17.
10. Landesman S, Jacard J, Gunderson V. The family environment: the combined influence of family behavior, goals, strategies, resources, and individual experiences. In: Lewis M, Feinman S, eds. *Social Influences on Development.* New York, NY: Plenum; 1991.
11. Bruner J. The organization of early skilled action. In: Richards MPM, ed. *The Integration of the Child Into a Social World.* New York, NY: Cambridge University Press; 1974.
12. Clarke-Stewart A. Interaction among mothers and their young children: characteristics and consequences. *Monogr Soc Res Child Dev.* 1973;38:6–7.
13. Tronick EZ, Gianino AF. The transmission of maternal disturbance to the infant. In: Tronick EZ, Field T, eds. *Maternal Depression and Infant Disturbance.* San Francisco, Calif: Jossey-Bass; 1986.
14. Slentz KL, Bricker D. Family-guided assessment for IFSP development: jumping off the family assessment bandwagon. *J Early Intervent.* 1992;16:1–19.
15. Bailey DB. Collaborative goal-setting with families: resolving differences in values and priorities for services. *Top Early Child Spec Educ.* 1987;7:59–71.
16. Johnson B, McGonigel M, Kaufmann R. *Guidelines and Recommended Practices for the Individualized Family Service Plan.* Chapel Hill, NC: National Early Childhood Technical Assistance System; 1989.
17. Kahn RJ. Brighter beginnings: a family centered/child focused mediated learning experience early intervention approach. Presented at DEC Sixth Annual International Early Childhood Conference on Children with Special Needs; Albuquerque, NM; October 20–24, 1990.
18. Dunst CJ, Trivette CM. An enablement and empowerment perspective of case management. *Top Early Child Spec Educ.* 1989;8:87–102.
19. Hausslein EB, Kaufmann RK, Hurth J. From case management to service coordination: families, policymaking, and Part H. *Zero to Three.* 1992;12:10–12.
20. Baskin C, Umansky W, Sanders W. Influencing the responsiveness of adolescent mothers to their infants. *Zero to Three.* 1987; 8:7–11.
21. Espe-Sherwindt M, Crable S. Parents with mental retardation: moving beyond the myths. *Top Early Child Spec Educ.* 1993;13:154–183.
22. Musick JS, Stott FM, Spencer KK, Goldman J, Cohler BJ. The capacity for "enabling" in mentally ill mothers. *Zero to Three.* 1984;4:1–6.
23. Bromwich RM. The interaction approach to early intervention. *Infant Mental Health J.* 1990;11:66–69.
24. Kahn RJ. Mediated learning experiences during parent/infant play interactions. *Int J Cogn Educ Med Learning.* 1992;2:131–146.
25. Winton PJ. Effective communication between parents and professionals. In: Bailey DB, Simeonsson RJ, eds. *Family Assessment in Early Intervention.* Columbus, Ohio: Merrill; 1988.

26. Carter SL, Osofsky JD, Hann DM. Speaking for the baby: a therapeutic intervention with adolescent mothers and their infants. *Infant Mental Health J.* 1991;12:291–301.
27. McCollum JA. At the crossroad: reviewing and rethinking interaction coaching. In: Marfo K, ed. *Early Intervention in Transition: Current Perspectives on Programs for Handicapped Children.* New York, NY: Praeger; 1991.
28. Beckwith L. Adaptive and maladaptive parenting: implications for intervention. In: Meisels S, Shonkoff J, eds. *Handbook of Early Childhood Intervention.* New York, NY: Cambridge University Press; 1990.
29. Isabella RA, Belsky J, von Eye A. Origins of infant-mother attachment: an examination of interactional synchrony during the infant's first year. *Dev Psychol.* 1989;25:12–21.
30. Kaye K. Organism, apprentice, and person. In: Tronick EZ, ed. *Social Interchange in Infancy: Affect, Cognition and Communication.* Baltimore, Md: University Park Press; 1982.
31. Goldberg S. Social competence in infancy: a model of parent-infant interaction. *Merrill-Palmer Q.* 1977;23:63–177.
32. Dunst CJ. Communicative competence and deficits: effects on early social interactions. In: McDonald ET, Gallagher DL, eds. *Facilitating Social-Emotional Development in Multiply-Handicapped Children.* Philadelphia, Pa: Michael C Prestegord; 1985.
33. Field T. The three Rs of infant-adult interactions: rhythms, repertoires, and responsivity. *J Pediatr Psychol.* 1978;3:131–136.
34. Field T. Interactions of high-risk infants: quantitative and qualitative differences. In: Sawin SB, Hawkins RC, Walker LO, Penticuff J, eds. *Exceptional Infant: Psychosocial Risks in Infant Environment Transactions.* New York, NY: Brunner/Mazel; 1980.
35. Cardone IA, Gilkerson L. Family administrated neonatal activities: an innovative component of family-centered care. *Zero to Three.* 1989;10:3–28.
36. Norton D. Understanding the early experience of black children in high risk environments: culturally and ecologically relevant research as a guide to support for families. *Zero to Three.* 1990;10:1–7.
37. Fraiberg S, Adelson E, Shapiro V. Ghosts in the nursery: a psychoanalytic approach to the problem of impaired infant-mother relationships. In: Fraiberg S, ed. *Clinical Studies in Infant Mental Health.* New York: Basic Books; 1980.
38. Kahn RJ. *Parents as Mediators of Their Children's Learning Experiences.* Final report, NIDRR innovation grant no. H133C90139. West Hartford, Conn: St Joseph College, Family Development Resource Center; 1990.
39. Kalmanson B, Seligman S. Family-provider relationships: the basis for all interventions. *Infants Young Child.* 1992;4:46–52.
40. Muir E. Watching, waiting, and wondering: applying psychoanalytic principles to mother-infant intervention. *Infant Mental Health J.* 1992;13:319–328.
41. Wieder S. Mediating successful parenting: guidelines for practitioners. *Zero to Three.* 1989;10:21–22.
42. Dunst C, Trivette C, Deal A. *Enabling and Empowering Families: Principles & Guidelines for Practice.* Cambridge, Mass: Brookline; 1988.
43. Wood D, Bruner JS, Ross G. The role of tutoring in problem solving. *J Child Psychol Psychiatry.* 1976;17:89–100.
44. McCollum JA, Bair H. Research in parent-child interaction: guidance to developmentally appropriate practice for young children with disabilities. In: Mallory B, New R, eds. *Diversity and*

Developmentally Appropriate Practice: Challenges for Early Childhood Education. New York, NY: Teachers College Press; 1993.

45. Musick JS, Bernstein V, Percansky C, Stott FM. A chain of enablement: using community-based programs to strengthen relationships between teen parents and their infants. *Zero to Three.* 1987;8:1–7.
46. Seitz V, Provence S. Caregiver-focused models of early intervention. In: Meisels SJ, Shonkoff JP, eds. *Handbook of Early Childhood Intervention.* Cambridge, England: Cambridge University Press; 1990.
47. Stern-Bruschweiler N, Stern DN. A model for conceptualizing the role of the mother's representational world in various mother-infant therapies. *Infant Mental Health J.* 1989;10:142–156.
48. Brown CW, Thorp EK. Individualizing training for early intervention practitioners. *Zero to Three.* 1989;10:8–12.
49. Fenichel E. Learning through supervision and mentorship to support the development of infants, toddlers and their families. *Zero to Three.* 1991;11:10–16.

Family-centered service coordination: A four-tier model

Ernestine E. Cormany, MA
Doctoral Candidate
Nova University
Fort Lauderdale, Florida
Child and Youth Studies Program/
Special Services
Chairperson
Brevard County Interagency
Community Collaboration Project
Cocoa, Florida

PUBLIC LAW 99-457, Part H (passed in 1986) and Public Law 102-119 (passed in 1991 to reenact Part H) have fundamentally altered policies and created new systems and subsystems of family-centered services for children with special needs and their families. Early intervention systems and their accompanying programs in all states have rapidly expanded since the passage of this legislation.[1,2] Through the use of federal "planning" dollars under Part H, states and local communities have actively engaged in developing comprehensive service delivery systems. This planning effort has sent policy makers, administrators, providers, and line staff scrambling for workable avenues to provide the core services necessary to comply with the law and move toward entitlement within the allotted time period in their respective states.

One of the most striking features of the new legislation is the family-centered approach and the core component requiring a "service coordinator" to assist in implementing the required Individualized Family Service Plan (IFSP). Over the generations, families have fought for a voice in structuring their child's care and education and for assistance in maneuvering through the complex and fragmented service delivery systems.[3–5] Proponents advocate for a skilled service coordinator as the key player in any efficient service system. A study of all 50 states and the District of Columbia showed that respondents believed that the service coordination portion of their early intervention system was the service area with the greatest need for reorganization and modification.[6]

Part H requires a service coordination system designed to create opportunities for integrated, community-based, family-centered services. It defines service coordination as activities carried out by a service coordinator to assist and enable eligible children and their families "to receive the rights, procedural safeguards and services that are authorized to be provided under the state's early intervention program."[7(p1)] Standards, certification, and licensing policies must be established and maintained for service coordinators. Service coordination must also be provided at no cost to parents.[8]

Historically, service coordination and case management emerged out of casework practices of social workers in the 1920s and 1930s and more recently from the deinstitutionalization movements in the mental health and mental retardation fields.[9,10] Contemporary service coordination practices have sprung up in response

Inf Young Children 1993; 6(2): 12–19

to the cry about fragmented and uncoordinated systems of human services and early intervention preschool programs. Initially the term "case management" was used to designate these services. Through public hearings and testimonies by parents and professionals who preferred not to have the negative connotation of being considered "cases" that needed to be "managed," the term "service coordination" was specifically endorsed in the PL 102-119 legislation. Because young children with special needs and their families often require comprehensive services that will unlikely come from any one agency, the legislation addresses the service coordination function and the service coordinator as the ultimate professional needed to "pull together" these services.

MODEL DEVELOPMENT

This article presents a four-tier model of service coordination for young children with special needs and their families. It was developed under a grant using Part H dollars and sponsored by the Florida Interagency Coordinating Council for Infants and Toddlers (FICCIT). The collaborative process was used from its inception. The article outlines the components of the model and presents the rationale for each component. The role and qualifications of the service coordinator in family-centered early intervention are also discussed as well as the benefits of the service coordination function.

The model is based on several assumptions about service coordination developed by parents and professionals and the megatrends affecting service delivery[3,9–12]:

- The role of the service coordinator is proactive with a shift from productivity measurement to quality of care.
- Service coordination should be family centered instead of system centered.
- Child and family concerns, priorities, and resources are recognized at the onset of service planning.
- Families are enabled and empowered through promoting family competencies to obtain resources and services.
- Families prefer a participatory democracy as opposed to a representative democracy.
- Family-centered service coordination is responsive to family concerns as well as to concerns related to children.
- Active efforts are necessary to avoid creating dependence or learned helplessness in families by teaching, encouraging, and reinforcing advocacy and independent decision-making skills.
- Families prefer a "one-stop-shopping" system of service coordination with one primary service coordinator to assist in coordinating their multiple service needs.

Based on these assumptions, and armed with the knowledge that a new design was needed to assure the delivery of quality services, an interagency collaborative effort was begun in a central Florida county to study the current problems and to design a workable model of effective service coordination.

INTERAGENCY DEVELOPMENT PROCESS

The first order of business for this project was to develop an understanding of the concept of a "collaborative" effort in contrast with a "cooperative" or "coordinating" effort.[13] If one were to place these concepts in a hierarchical framework (Fig 1), the cooperative phase would represent the lowest rung on the totem pole. Although very important, this cooperative effort merely represents a feeling of peaceful coexistence with agencies working informally together in a loosely defined and unstructured arrangement.

Next would come the phase of coordination. The coordination effort provides a more formalized effort of teamwork with agencies working jointly to schedule activities and plan for services for designated groups of children. Last would be the highest level of interagency planning and activity, the collaborative effort. The collaborative effort shows previously separate and independent functions working in synch. These functions become a new unit with a mutual goal. The joint problem solving, sharing, and merging of resources subsequently leads to the creation of new programs. This project saw a natural evolution in this hierarchy with the final product of a service coordination model developed through a collaborative effort.

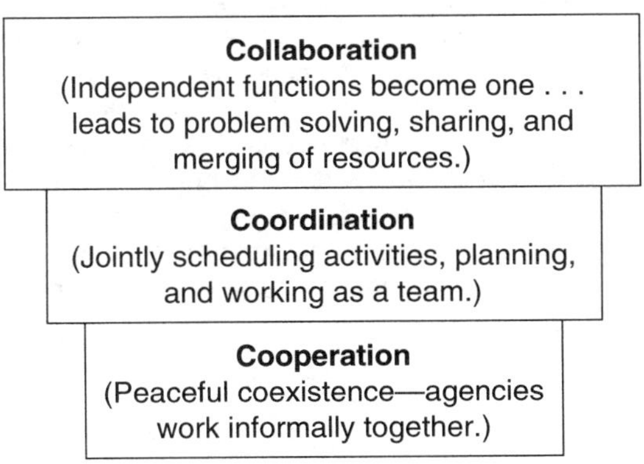

Fig 1. Hierarchical design representative of the community interagency planning process. Adapted with permission from the Bureau of Education for Exceptional Students, Division of Public Schools, Florida Department of Education.

CASE EXAMPLE

The following case example illustrates the need for a workable service coordination model as intended under Part H guidelines.

Jerry and Jill Davis (not their real names) are the parents of a 7-month-old daughter, Sarah. Sarah was born with Down syndrome, a heart defect, and visual impairments. Jerry and Jill have one other child, Jason, who is 4 years old. He appears to be very bright and attends a private preschool.

Jerry, an engineer with a promising future, is completing the last semester of a master's in business administration program at a local university. He has become quiet and withdrawn since Sarah was born, has often questioned the genetic underpinnings of Sarah's birth, and has engaged in self-blaming behaviors.

Jill worked as a public relations officer for a large corporation associated with the space industry prior to Sarah's birth. She took a 3-month leave of absence to be at home with the new infant. Even with Jill's high energy level, bubbly personality, and commitment to follow every service system lead possible to secure services for Sarah she is beginning to show signs of stress and defeat. Marital discord, frequent headaches, concerns regarding Jason's behavior in preschool, and financial problems have led Jill to question how much longer she can continue at this pace.

Initially the Davis family had not been sure where to turn when their pediatrician announced a few hours after Sarah's birth that there were "complications." This announcement was followed by countless hours, days, and weeks of pursuing possible service leads and repeating Sarah's "story." Jill called or visited the state developmental services agency, the supplemental security income (SSI) office, the school system's Child Find program, the health department, the children's medical services office for genetic counseling, the Association for Retarded Citizens (ARC), the ophthalmologist, the cardiologist, and countless others. With each contact, program case managers or service coordinators, social workers, nurse practitioners, and other allied professionals asked the same questions and were assigned to her "case."

Jill's frustration became evident when she finally broke down in a visit to her personal physician who recommended counseling and therapy sessions for her and her husband. One more appointment . . . one more thing to work into her schedule. Jill wanted and needed to return to her job. She had been able to enroll Sarah in the ARC early intervention program for morning programming and in a day care center for afternoon care. She needed help to arrange for transportation—one more hurdle to overcome.

Jerry and Jill's story is commonplace, not atypical. The fragmented, complex, and outdated service delivery system is contributing to the already overwhelming concerns of this family. The following four-tier model (Fig 2) is presented to address the letter of the law as intended in PL 99-457 and PL 102-119 and is offered as a method for improving outcomes for children and their families as they seek services. Additional benefits are provided in the clear-cut roles given to service providers and the ultimate cost effectiveness of this approach.

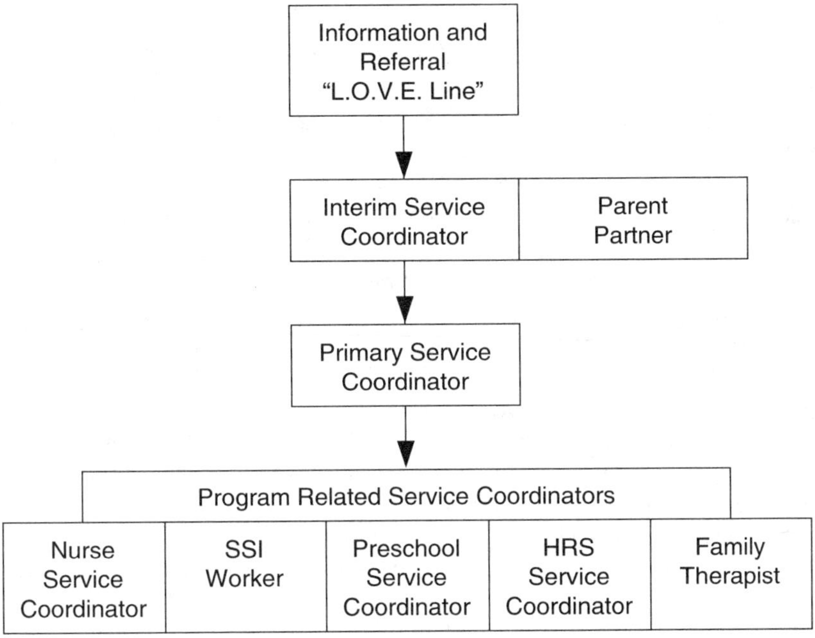

Fig 2. The four-tier model of service coordination for young children with special needs and their families. SSI = supplemental security income; HRS = health and rehabilitative services.

MODEL DESIGN

Tier 1, the Information and Referral "L.O.V.E. Line," is designed to be an initial contact point for families, physicians, and other providers. This Local Outreach for Varying Exceptionalities (L.O.V.E.) line represents a "one-stop-shopping" entry into the system and is accessed by one toll-free telephone number. This simulated information bank is staffed by sensitive personnel who answer questions and gather basic information regarding the child and family in order to initiate services. A preliminary assessment is made in this first tier to determine the crisis or noncrisis nature of the call. Calls of a crisis nature are immediately channeled to a long-established crisis hotline serving the county.

Noncrisis calls requesting services for children with special needs and their families are directed to the tier 2 Interim Service Coordinator. This Interim Service Coordinator is required to make a personal contact with the family within 2 days of the original call to the L.O.V.E. line. An intake meeting (using a countywide mutually agreed on intake instrument through the collaborative process) is arranged. The purpose of the intake meeting is for information gathering and screening and the assignment of a parent partner through family choice. To assure the timely delivery of services as required by Part H,[14] the service inquiry is processed through tier 2 in a maximum of 45 days, concluding with the IFSP meeting. During this 45-day period, evaluations of child and family concerns, priorities, and resources take place and appropriate linkages for initial services are made. The first IFSP meeting is scheduled and facilitated by the Interim Service Coordinator, and the assignment of a Primary Service Coordinator at the IFSP meeting signals the move to tier 3 of the model.

The Primary Service Coordinator provides a single point of contact for families[15,16] and holds primary responsibility for the implementation and coordination of all services.[6] The Primary Service Coordinator is viewed as the worker for the family, not for any particular agency. A generalist approach to the job responsibilities of the Primary Service Coordinator incorporates the coordination and monitoring of services across various service providers[9] and the planning and integration of all resources and supports.[14,17]

Seven benefits of the primary service coordination system include a provision for

1. families to receive relevant information in a more convenient manner,
2. families to learn more about additional services to meet their needs,
3. lessening of the demands on families to travel to many sites and repeat the same information,
4. families to develop a trusting relationship with a single professional and a means for receiving the training necessary to become empowered and take more control over their own lives,
5. service systems to eliminate the costly duplication of services,
6. a more effective system of documentation and accountability, and
7. a mechanism for feeding information back to service delivery systems and funding sources for future planning and needs identification.

It is the responsibility of the team developing the IFSP to determine who will serve as the Primary Service Coordinator. In some states independent service coordination organizations, free of agency ties, have been set up to handle the Primary Service Coordinator's responsibilities.[15,18] The model presented in this article, however, draws on service coordinators in the county's provider agencies to serve in these primary roles. Because of the special tasks involved in coordination across agency lines this approach presents a special challenge. It has been essential to establish effective partnerships and collaborative relationships between all involved in the early intervention process in order to make this a workable model. The approval and support of agency heads have been paramount in setting aside loyalty to particular agencies and disciplines.[7]

When designating a Primary Service Coordinator, two important considerations are the profession most relevant to the needs of the child and family and the choice of the family. The IFSP team assesses the abilities and workloads of the individuals under consideration.[14] The intensity, duration, and complexity of the service needs are also evaluated. While in many instances there is a real need for a professional to assist the children and families as Primary Service Coordinator, it is also important to give credit to those families who may wish to play a major role in coordinating their own services. This option may be seen as an ever-increasing possibility as professionals work to empower families, create positive self-sufficiency, teach assertive and advocacy behaviors, and impart independent decision-making skills.

Tier 4 of the model represents a subset of the primary service coordination system, referred to as Program-Related Service Coordinators. The Program-Related Service Coordinator's role is reminiscent of the most common type of case management/service coordination in most service systems today. A review of the literature [15,18,19] shows that program-related service coordination focuses primarily on specific needs of consumers based on eligibility and program priorities. This system involves rationing services in some "direct" manner by matching consumer needs, vendor priorities, and available funding.

Recognizing that this link is important in planning for services, Primary Service Coordinators and families continue to need the participation of Program-Related Service Coordinators in: (1) initial and annual IFSP meetings as deemed appropriate, (2) the provision of information regarding available service options and eligibility criteria for their respective programs, (3) the provision of information on enrollment procedures, payment authorization, and voucher completion for specific services, (4) the maintenance of program-specific consumer files, and (5) the completion of required legal forms and documentation relative to programmatic concerns.[20] Under this model, families continue to maintain a certain amount of contact with Program-Related Service Coordinators. Based on the most prevalent needs of children and families one of the Program-Related Service Coordinators will more than likely be designated as the Primary Service Coordinator under this model.

In the scenario presented in the case study, the Davis family would have no doubt benefited from this four-tier model of family-centered service coordination. Moreover, the scenario would probably have been quite different. Although a vast improvement over previous service delivery, the model should not be considered a panacea for curing all the ills related to the developmental disabilities service system. The model does, however, provide a much needed framework to assist families in the complex and fragmented process of accessing services.

ROLES, RESPONSIBILITIES, AND TRAINING OF CASE MANAGERS

In order for this model or any other model to work, an important component must be addressed: adequate training of all service coordination staff members.[11,12] Service coordinators must be steeped in both practice and systems knowledge regarding infant and toddler development, PL 99-457 (Part H) and PL 102-119 and their regulations, early intervention service systems, and funding sources and the mechanics necessary to access them.[21] Service coordinators must also learn to be positive and proactive in interactions with families, permitting families to decide whether to accept or reject help,[22] and possess the ability to avoid labeling and blaming behaviors. Implications for service coordination practice also indicate that all front-line service coordinators need clear guidelines about the amount of time they are expected to spend with consumers, specific standards for the focus and content of child and family objectives, and well-defined goals.[23,24] Various studies[7,10,11,14] of individuals serving in early intervention service coordination roles indicate that social workers, nurses, educators, and therapists are among the most common professions represented.

Because the role of service coordinator may be seen as that of listener, consultant, resource, enabler, mobilizer, mediator, advocate, cost accountant, and facilitator, specialized training is a must. With the anticipated growth of early intervention programs, colleges and universities may be forced into helping students become better prepared across all disciplines to deal with the demands of their future positions. Training service coordinators to be well versed in financial and technologic areas is becoming increasingly more important. In many cases, estimating the costs of care plans, negotiating service rates with providers, and using information systems to track clients are skills rivaling those previously considered necessary in social service delivery. A progressive approach toward independent study and group study may also be advocated in order to keep pace with future projections. Service coordination certification examinations and continuing education units (CEUs) necessary for annual renewal are currently being considered.[7]

• • •

Although early intervention practices and the family-centered approach have come a long way in a short period of time, many challenges continue to lie ahead. It is a well-known fact that all children, with or without special needs, need their families. It is also well known that families who are getting their own needs met are better able to meet the needs of their children.

The rigid uniformity on the one hand and the lackadaisical disregard for underservice or overservice on the other are hopefully things of the past. Recognizing that the presenting needs of consumers require varying depths, designs, and intensities of service coordination should lead to operating models that are need responsive, time and cost efficient, and outcome productive. Service coordination does not exist in a vacuum. We must be forever mindful that without direct services for children and their families, service coordinators would have no resources or systems to coordinate. Every effort must be made to continue adequate funding and support for quality social services consistent with guiding values and principles and environmental requirements and constraints.

It is imperative that effective family-centered service coordination programs improve the quality of life for children with special needs and their families. This improvement will be accomplished by strengthening individual opportunities, increasing self determination, and expanding personal choice and responsibility. The empowerment of families fostered through learning needed skills has in itself a well-documented payoff. Keeping children and families together is one of life's most precious rewards. The cost savings provided to taxpayers through lessening residential and institutional placements of developmentally disabled children must also be acknowledged.

The federal government in its infinite wisdom has provided a framework for program development under PL 99-457 and PL 102-119. These laws allow states and local communities to plan for and develop ownership of their own early intervention service system design. The four-tier model for family-centered service coordination presented in this article represents one such practical and workable model built on the local community collaboration process.

REFERENCES

1. Bailey DB, Buysse V, Edmondson R, Smith TM. Creating family-centered services in early intervention: perceptions of professionals in four states. *Except Child.* 1992;58:298–309.
2. Krauss MW. New precedent in family policy: individualized family service plan. *Except Child.* 1990;56:388–395.
3. Austin CD. Case management: myths and realities. *Families in Society: J Contemporary Human Services.* 1990;51:398–405.
4. Meisels SJ, Harbin G, Modigliani K, Olson K. Formulating optimal state early intervention policies. *Except Child.* 1988;55:159–165.
5. Turnbull R, Turnbull A. Including all children. *Child Today.* 1991;20:3–5.
6. Bureau of Education for Exceptional Students, Division of Public Schools. *Interagency Problem Solving.* Tallahassee, Fla: Florida Department of Education; 1989.
7. Florida Department of Education. *Proposed Case Management System for Serving Florida* (Phase II Findings). Tallahassee, Fla: Florida State University, Policy Studies Clinic, College of Law and The Center for Prevention and Early Intervention Policy; 1991.
8. Ballard J, Ramirez B, Zantal-Wiener K. *Public Law 94-142, Section 504, and Public Law 99-457: Understanding What They Are and Are Not.* Reston, Va: The Council for Exceptional Children; 1989.
9. Dunst CJ, Trivette CM. An enablement and empowerment perspective on case management. *Top Early Child Spec Ed.* 1988;8:87–102.
10. Fiene JI, Taylor PA. Serving rural families of developmentally disabled children: a case management model. *Soc Work.* 1991;36:323–327.

11. Bailey DB, Palsha SA, Simeonsson RJ. Professional skills, concerns, and perceived importance of work with families in early intervention. *Except Child.* 1991;58:156–163.
12. Dunst CJ, Johanson C, Trivette CM, Hamby D. Family-oriented early intervention policies and practices: family-centered or not? *Except Child.* 1991;58:115–125.
13. Bureau of Education for Exceptional Students, Division of Public Schools. *A Rationale for Interagency Collaboration.* Tallahassee, Fla: Florida Department of Education; 1991.
14. Duwa S. *The Family Support Plan Process* (Module 1: Participants Manual). Tallahassee, Fla: Florida State University Center for Prevention and Early Intervention; 1992.
15. Florida Developmental Disabilities Planning Council and State of Florida. *Consumer and Family Access to Services: An Integrated Model for Case Management* (Final Report). Tallahassee, Fla: Department of Health and Rehabilitative Services; 1991.
16. Parent Resource Organization. *Best Practices for the Four Core Services.* Tallahassee, Fla: PRO; 1992.
17. Tracy EM. Identifying social support resources of at-risk families. *Soc Work.* 1990;35:252–257.
18. Florida Department of Education. *Thirteen Models of Case Management.* (Cost/implementation study for PL 99-457; Policy Studies Clinic). Tallahassee, Fla: Florida State University, College of Law; 1992.
19. Karp N, Bradley V. A state of the states: family support. *Child Today.* 1991;20:28–31.
20. Metz IB, Hoot JL. *Crossroads: Cooperative Transagency Program for Preschool Culturally/Linguistically Diverse Exceptional Children.* Washington, DC: US Depart of Education; 1990. ERIC Document Reproduction Service no. ED 340 192.
21. United Cerebral Palsy Associations. *Family Focused Early Intervention.* Washington, DC: US Depart of Education; 1992.
22. Dunst CJ, Trivette CM, Deal AG. *Enabling and Empowering Families: Principles and Guidelines for Practice.* Cambridge, Mass: Brookline; 1988.
23. Ronnau JP. A strengths approach to helping family caregiver. *Child Today.* 1992;19:24–27.
24. Garland C. *Case Management.* (Division for Early Childhood White Paper). Birmingham, England: Association of Workers for Maladjusted Children; 1988. ERIC Document Reproduction Service no. ED 300 940.

Infants and young children with HIV infection: Service delivery considerations for family support

Sharon Lesar, PhD
Center for Family Studies
Western Carolina Center
Morganton, North Carolina

Yvonne A. Maldonado, MD
Department of Pediatrics
Stanford University School of Medicine
Stanford, California

INCREASING numbers of children are being diagnosed with the human immunodeficiency virus (HIV) infection. As of October 1992, about 4,051 acquired immunodeficiency syndrome (AIDS) cases in children under 13 years of age had been reported to the Centers for Disease Control (CDC). The number of perinatally infected infants nearly doubled compared with the previous year. However, because the CDC uses rigid criteria for classifying AIDS cases and many cases of pediatric AIDS are mistaken for other immune disorders, experts estimate that for every child reported to have AIDS, 2 to 10 children may be HIV infected.[1] Although there is no national count of HIV-infected individuals, it is estimated that between 7,575 and 17,675 children are HIV infected. Thus, this current epidemic is becoming a disease of children that has tragic consequences not only for infected children, but also for their parents, families, and communities. Moreover, these estimates may be interpreted to suggest a dramatic increase in demand for early intervention and related services for children and their families.

Typically, most children with HIV infection have or will acquire significant developmental delays or loss of developmental achievement as a result of the affect of the virus on the central nervous system.[2] HIV infection of the central nervous system may eventually produce a progressive encephalopathy, which results in neuropathologic abnormalities in cognitive, motor, linguistic, psychosocial, and sensory/perceptual development.[3,4] The wide range of developmental disabilities or neuromuscular dysfunction associated with HIV infection poses a significant dilemma for those planning or providing services for young children with HIV infection. Children with HIV infection may have special education needs and are eligible for enrollment in an early intervention program under the Individuals with Disabilities Education Act (IDEA). Moreover, children with HIV infection who are at risk for developmental disabilities because of an established condition but whose development is not yet sufficiently significantly delayed to meet established criteria for eligibility need services as well. (Head Start is an example of a program that works on this principle.)

SUPPORT FOR FAMILY CAREGIVERS

Care for young children diagnosed with HIV presents extraordinary medical, psychological, and financial demands that can be expected to strain the caretaking

Inf Young Children 1994; 6(4): 70–81

capabilities of any family, thereby raising concerns about the children's welfare and the impact their illness has on families. This has created unique challenges to service providers in understanding the difficulties of coping with AIDS, particularly for families who have young children with HIV, and in providing information and services to address their varied needs.

The stress caused by HIV in families can be devastating. Individual responses to HIV vary with basic coping abilities and physical health; availability of support from family, friends, and others; concrete resources; the degree of illness; and spiritual strengths and beliefs.[5] Changes in the child's behavior, physical needs, and mental abilities also affect the stress level experienced by caregivers. The HIV-infected child can be limited physically, psychologically, and socially in mastering the stages of development.[2,6,7] At a time when children are expected to become more autonomous, self-initiating, and capable, the HIV-infected child is faced with an illness that renders him or her dependent, vulnerable, and often helpless.[8] An estimated 20% to 40% of HIV-infected children now require foster or group home placement, often because birth families are too overwhelmed by their own illness and lack the ability or resources to continue providing care for them. The purpose of this article is to describe the family adaptational model for HIV-infected children and to present initial findings from our research that have implications for service providers. Service delivery considerations for family support are discussed in terms of helping families adjust and adapt to pediatric HIV infection.

A FAMILY SYSTEMS ADAPTATIONAL MODEL

Family system theory encompasses the fundamental tenets of both ecological and social network theories,[9–14] in that ecological units do not operate in isolation but interact both within and between levels, so that changes in one unit or subunit reverberate and impact on other units. Thus a specific stressor reverberates through a family and has both direct and indirect influences on family members. Within the context of providing care to children with HIV infection, it is imperative that the child be considered as part of a total family system. For every child with perinatal HIV infection, there is a mother with infection and possibly a father who is ill. Therefore, any comprehensive model must treat the child as part of a family unit, and this family must be recognized as having its own needs independent of direct services to the child.

Despite the acknowledged importance of the immediate "family" of the HIV-infected child, relatively little research has examined the relevant family processes related to basic developmental achievements in meeting physical, social, and cognitive milestones, or how these processes are affected by parental social support and the ongoing social, economic, and psychological demands placed on the family system. We have been engaged in both clinical and research efforts designed to learn more about the impact on and complexities of family functioning and adaptation in young children with HIV infection. This work has culminated in the development of a conceptual framework that integrates the concepts of stress, coping, and ecological systems into a single model with which to investigate and understand the impact of children with HIV infection on family systems. This model draws theoretical and empirical information from a number of extant conceptual frameworks, including specifically Bronfenbrenner's[15] discussion of the importance of ecological variables to familial functioning and the impact of the child's chronic illness on parents, siblings, and extended family members; McCubbin and Patterson's[16] Double ABCX model of family adjustment and adaptation; and Dunst et al's[17] social systems model of family functioning. The family adaptational model is presented in schematic form in Fig 1.

We conducted a study with 48 family caregivers of HIV-exposed children in northern and central California to empirically examine the family adaptational model. These caregivers were birth parents, extended family members, or foster parents responsible for the care of the child. Caregivers were recruited with letters and flyers sent by staff at two of the northern California pediatric AIDS treatment centers or by service providers at AIDS agencies that work with families. To control for the effects of risk factors other than HIV infection, uninfected infants and children with perinatal HIV exposure served as a control population to the HIV-infected group.

Demographic characteristics of the caregivers, as well as information about their HIV-exposed children, are presented in Table 1. Of the mothers infected with HIV, 35% were exposed to the virus through intravenous (IV) needle sharing, 31% through a sexual partner of unknown risk, 13% through a sexual partner who was an IV drug user, and 6% through unknown exposure. Thirty-three percent of the HIV-exposed children had some type of developmental delay; however, 45% of the HIV-infected children (N = 31) had developmental delays. These developmental disabilities were in the areas of cognitive impairments, deficits in both gross and fine motor skills, language delays, and loss of developmental milestones.

The caregivers completed the following four self-report questionnaires and one audiotaped semistructured face-to-face interview as part of their participation in the study: Family Support Scale,[18] Coping Health Inventory for Parents,[19] Impact on Family Scale,[20] Questionnaire on Resources and Stress,[21] and the Impact on Caregiver Personal Interview (Lesar S, unpublished scale, Stanford University School of Medicine, 1993). These measures collected both qualitative and quantitative data on parenting stress, social support, coping behaviors, and the impact of a chronically ill child on family functioning. We used a multidimensional approach to examine how child characteristics, social support, adequacy of resources, and coping styles relate to family outcomes in families of HIV-infected children. The following discussion is based on the data generated from the interviews as it relates to family adaptation and functioning.

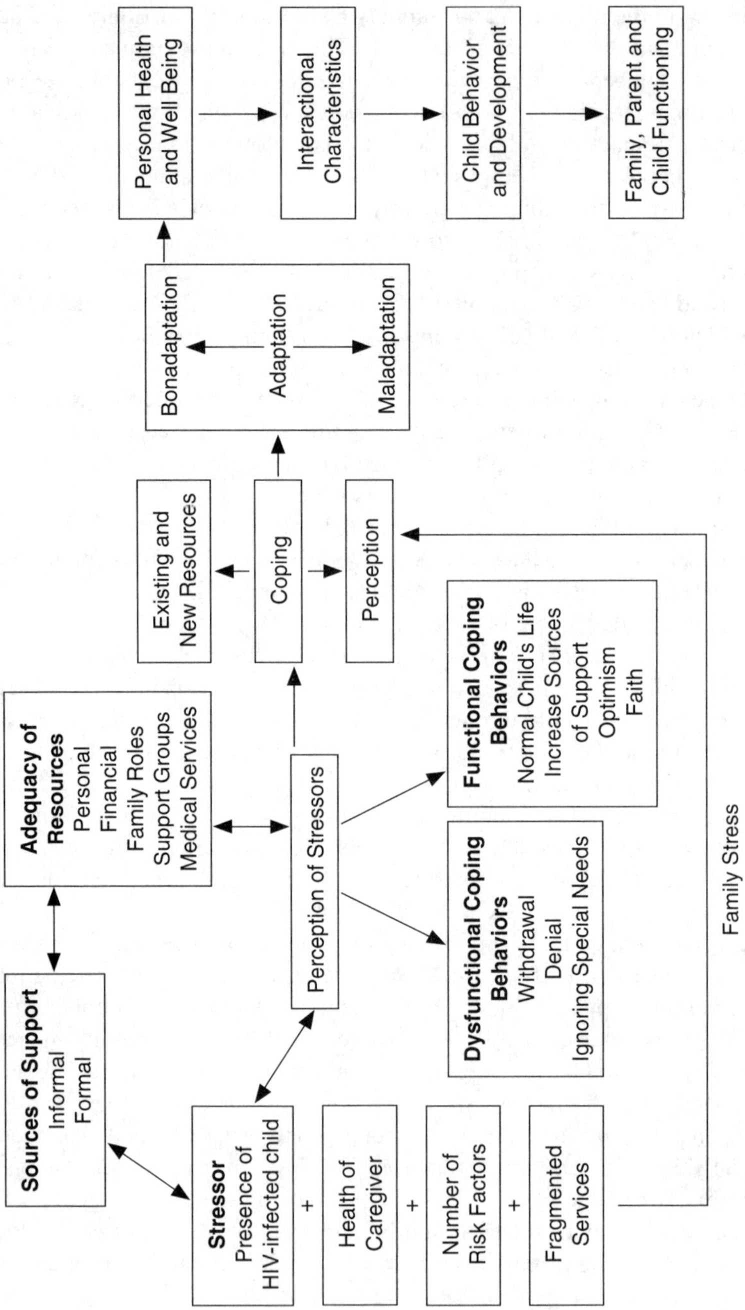

Fig 1. Family adaptational model for families with an HIV-infected child.

Table 1. Study sample characteristics (N = 48)

Variable	HIV Positive		HIV Negative		Total	
	%	(n)	%	(n)	%	(n)
Child characteristics						
HIV status						
HIV asymptomatic	9.7	(3)			6.3	(3)
HIV symptomatic	90.3	(28)			58.3	(28)
Indeterminate					10.4	(5)
Seroreverter			100	(12)	25.0	(12)
Gender						
Male	41.9	(13)	50.0	(6)	44.8	(21)
Female	58.1	(18)	50.0	(6)	56.2	(27)
Ethnicity						
African American	51.6	(16)	66.6	(8)	54.2	(26)
White	32.3	(10)	16.7	(2)	27.1	(13)
Hispanic	12.9	(4)	16.7	(2)	14.6	(7)
Asian					2.1	(1)
American Indian					2.1	(1)
HIV transmission						
Mother with HIV risk	77.4	(24)	100	(12)	85.4	(41)
Pediatric hemophilia	6.5	(2)			4.2	(2)
Pediatric transfusion	16.1	(5)			10.4	(5)
Caregiver characteristics						
HIV status						
HIV asymptomatic	38.7	(12)	25.0	(3)	20.8	(10)
HIV symptomatic			41.7	(5)	29.2	(14)
HIV negative	61.3	(19)	33.3	(4)	50.0	(24)
Ethnicity						
African American	35.5	(11)	58.3	(7)	39.6	(19)
White	51.6	(16)	41.7	(5)	47.9	(23)
Hispanic	9.7	(3)			8.3	(4)
Asian	3.2	(1)			2.1	(1)
American Indian					2.1	(1)
Marital status						
Married	35.5	(11)	41.7	(5)	41.7	(20)
Single	64.5	(20)	58.3	(7)	58.3	(28)
Employment						
Working full time	12.9	(4)	8.3	(1)	10.4	(5)
Currently not working	87.1	(27)	91.7	(11)	89.6	(43)
Income level						
Under $12,000	25.8	(8)	58.3	(7)	35.4	(17)
$12,000–$21,000	35.5	(11)	8.3	(1)	29.2	(14)
$21,000–$30,000	19.4	(6)	8.3	(1)	14.6	(7)
Over $30,000	19.4	(6)	25.0	(3)	20.8	(10)
Source of income						
Salary/income	35.5	(11)	25.0	(3)	33.3	(16)
Entitlements: AFDC, Social Security	54.8	(17)	66.7	(8)	56.3	(27)
Other	9.7	(3)	8.3	(1)	10.4	(5)
Relationship to child						
Birthparent	64.5	(20)	66.7	(8)	66.7	(32)
Relative	12.9	(4)	8.3	(1)	10.4	(5)
Foster/adoptive parent	22.6	(7)	25.0	(3)	22.9	(11)

Many of the families in this study reported that they had adapted successfully to the sustained, stressful experiences associated with their child's condition and prolonged interactions with the health care system. As the families were interviewed, they seemed to describe a remarkably uniform adaptation to life with a young child with HIV infection, based on the family adaptational model.

At first, caregivers were overwhelmed and despondent about their perception of their child's HIV status. Some caregivers withdrew from social involvement or coped by denying the reality of their child's diagnosis. Others initiated aggressive searches of support and services for their child or tried to bring about societal changes that would be more supportive of families with HIV-infected children. Slowly, these parents began to learn about the health care system and to evaluate the care provided to their child. They began to gather information for themselves and to gain skills and knowledge related to their child's care. These families struggled to achieve a fit at both the individual-to-family and the family-to-community levels by accessing available resources and social support.

The appraisal of stressors and of their capabilities to manage required many families to use new resources, as well as coping and problem-solving efforts. For example, to cope with their frustration and anger, some families became involved in HIV educational training in the community, public speaking at schools, and the National Pediatric AIDS Foundation. One family explained that "the educational process has been one of the key elements for both of us for working out that frustration." The majority of the caregivers indicated that they are a closer family because of what they have shared.

As these families struggle to cope with the diagnosis of HIV and other stressors in their environment, family system adjustment occurs and, over time, achieves some level of adaptation. These families may be adaptive in their functioning when examined within the broader context of the child's condition and care. The findings from our study empirically support the family adaptational model as a theoretical framework for understanding the impact of pediatric HIV on the family system. Specifically, the influence of the child's developmental and HIV status, the caregiver's HIV status, and caregiving demands on family stress was supported by results of statistical analyses. However, types and sources of support were not significantly related to caregivers' stress ratings. The data provided evidence that types of support are significantly linked to caregivers' HIV status and children's developmental delay status.

We have selected three aspects of our findings to utilize in discussing the model's application to work with families: the influences of both formal and informal social support, the availability of services and unmet services needs, and the implications for service providers. To illustrate our findings, selected case material will be presented. Direct quotations from the interviews are presented, with clarifying contextual material added.

Social support

Contrary to previous research, social support did not have a buffering effect on reducing stress in our study. This could be due to the stigmatization and isolation of the disease. This is further substantiated by the personal interviews conducted with the caregivers. Seventy percent of the caregivers reported telling only their immediate family about their HIV diagnosis for fear of misunderstanding and stigma attached to HIV. Thus, the interaction of the caregiver with others in her social world is altered because of the social stigma of HIV, as well as the child's chronic illness. Consider the following case of a family with HIV:

> And then there were people that were . . . they threw things at me. They cussed me out. They threatened my life and my family. It was pretty crazy. At one time these people broke into my sister's house [where they were living] and destroyed everything. It wasn't about theft. It was about hate.

When these caregivers were asked how they decided who to tell or not tell, they said that they felt that they wanted to tell their immediate family, but they kept it from friends, neighbors, and other people because of their fear of their reactions. Many of the families reported being stigmatized by family relatives, friends, church members, child-care providers, and medical staff. Thus, different types of social support were not significantly helpful in caring for an HIV-exposed child.

In addition, the results indicate that HIV-positive caregivers, compared with their HIV-negative counterparts, received significantly less total social support and informal social support. This finding further confirms that families with HIV do not rely on their social support network because of their fear of rejection, social isolation, feelings of guilt and shame, and the stigma attached to an HIV diagnosis. However, caregivers of children who had developmental delays received significantly more total social support and immediate family support.

The findings indicate that specific sources of support are elicited by the caregiver's HIV status and the child's developmental delay status. These findings suggest that social support does not directly influence well-being but does have indirect influences on child characteristics, which in turn may influence family well-being. For example, the various sources of social support may have a buffering effect on families raising a young HIV-infected child with developmental delays. Therefore, interventions aimed at providing support and resources to families caring for HIV-exposed children can be expected to have "second-order" influences on buffering stress. Thus, there are several plausible theories that can explain the relationships among social support, parenting stress, and pediatric HIV.

There are many illustrations of the indirect influences of social support on this cohort of families. One example of the indirect influence of social support can be illustrated through the story of Mrs. R, a foster mother who expressed concern, grief, and frustration over her 3-year-old daughter's AIDS status. When asked what she did to help her daughter and herself cope with AIDS, Mrs. R said that she often talks with the medical staff at the pediatric HIV clinic. In addition, Mrs. R participates in a foster parent group for medically fragile children, where she talks with other parents about her fears and frustrations and shares medical information. When her daughter's illness becomes "too much to handle," Mrs. R asks her husband to babysit for a while to give her a break. These support resources clearly provide Mrs. R with a range of emotional, informational, and instrumental support. However, when Mrs. R was asked what kinds of help were most useful, she responded, "Just the understanding, just knowing I can get help when I need it."

The social stigma attached to HIV infection may be another plausible reason why social support did not insulate these families from stress. In response to the social stigma of the disease, one mother said "I would prefer that everybody would be able to know and not have a problem, but I didn't want my son to get any backlash from it." The stigma and burdens associated with HIV infection are unique. Caregivers suffer great guilt and anger about transmitting the disease to their children. All of the HIV-infected mothers in this study worried about what would happen to their children when they were no longer around. In many ways, these families have less community support than do adult HIV victims who are homosexual. They have less peer group identity than do homosexual men and, subsequently, less support in the HIV experience.

Although some of the families and children in our study were open about their diagnosis, most families kept it a well-guarded secret. Families often kept the diagnosis a secret in order to maintain a sense of normalcy in their lives. One caregiver described her family's sensitivity about HIV in this way:

> I would like them to know that we are normal people. The sickness that we have in our family is something that we take care of. We don't try to push it on anyone, or hope that no one comes along and gets the sickness that is in the family, but we would love to be continued to be treated like a normal family.

For this family and others, the sense of being treated no differently than others was a common thread. Even though these families have at least one family member with HIV, they appear to have adapted and adjusted to the diagnosis. Further educational efforts must be made to reduce the stigma of HIV and the discrimination against and isolation of families with HIV infection.

Availability of services and unmet service needs

Another area we addressed was the services available to help the family system cope with a young child infected with HIV. The responses from the personal interview elicited the types of services available and unmet service needs. For the most part, hospitals, medical providers, and AIDS agencies provide the majority of services to this population. The array of services vary according to where the caregiver resides and which treatment center is providing medical services to the child.

Caregivers reported finding these services either by seeking them out on their own or through hospital treatment centers. Some families felt frustrated because they did not really know what types of services were available to them or how to access them. Caregivers who attended either a monthly support group at one of the medical treatment centers or foster parent support groups reported finding out about local services from other parents who were caring for HIV-infected children. Caregivers who attended these support groups felt that the opportunity to talk to other families experiencing the same circumstances was supportive, helping them feel that they were not alone in this disease. However, only one of the treatment centers and one of the county medically fragile foster parent programs had support groups, thus limiting accessibility for families caring for HIV-infected children.

Even though a variety of services were available to these families, many felt frustrated because of the limitation of the services. Depending on which county the caregiver resides in, respite care is often not provided for foster parents and is only provided to other families if there is a volunteer agency that provides respite care for HIV-infected children. The majority of families who lived in San Francisco received some type of respite care from the Shanti Project, a nonprofit volunteer AIDS agency, or funds provided through foster care. Families living in other areas received little or no respite care.

Ninety-six percent of the caregivers felt that the services they received were helpful; however, many felt that the services were limited in certain aspects. For example, one caregiver complained that

> Like any other support group, they meet only once a month, so if you have a problem you better work it out before the end of the month because you have lost your cause. There needs to be something more available to people so when the problem arises you can talk to somebody about it right away.

In addition, many of the volunteers who provide respite care are not allowed to administer medication, can stay for a maximum of only 4 hours, or have different time schedules that often do not coincide with the caregivers' needs. One caregiver described this frustration by saying

> They don't want to work on weekends. They don't want to work Friday night so you can go out. They want to come Thursday afternoon from 2 to 4 and you have nowhere to go.

Another consistent finding that emerged from the interviews was the inability to access reliable child care. This was particularly true when caregivers chose to disclose their child's HIV status. All of the caregivers who disclosed their child's HIV status to child-care programs were denied access initially. Thus, some of these mothers had to quit their jobs to care for their child because they could not find child care. Medical professionals and child-care coordinating agencies often advised these caregivers not to disclose their child's HIV status because of the stigma attached to the disease. However, 36% of the caregivers decided to disclose their child's HIV status because they were concerned about their child being exposed to other children's infections. One mother reported that

> It took me 6 weeks to find him day care. I didn't have a day care so I had friends taking care of him on different days so that I could keep my job. The child care I initially found kept him in a crib in a room by himself and he was not allowed to socialize with other children. But I didn't have anywhere else to take him.

Other caregivers have had to pave the way for other families to obtain child-care services. One mother described how she initially placed her son in a preschool program without telling the program's administrators about his diagnosis. Later she told them of his HIV status and how they could not deny him access because of the Americans with Disabilities Act. Other caregivers had to provide HIV education training for all child-care staff in order to enlist their child in the program.

Of the HIV-infected children who had developmental delays, more than 70% received some type of early intervention or special education services. The majority of the caregivers reported that they had to seek out and demand these services for their children. When asked how they found out about these services, most caregivers said that they had to find out on their own, either by calling agencies or talking to other people. One father recalled his experience of finding out about early intervention services:

> I didn't find out about the regional center until my son was almost 2½ years old. Where I specifically found out about it, I don't remember. It may have been my health insurance company asking me why I don't have this going on.

Compare this perspective with that of a foster parent who had taken care of other HIV-infected foster children:

> I guess I just knew from experience. The infant program came through the regional center and I knew about it too. It was all stuff I had known about in the past. Most of the time we are the ones educating the social workers. We are the ones with the knowledge but they are the ones with the power.

Thus, in many instances, many of these children with developmental delays received limited or delayed services. This is alarming, as all of these children were regularly seen by pediatricians, social workers, and, often, child development psychologists.

Implications for service providers

Children who suffer from chronic or terminal illnesses other than HIV are encouraged to strive for as normal a life as possible. The goal should be the same for a child with HIV infection. However, emotions and fears are stirred when a child with HIV pursues a normal life by attempting to attend day care or preschool.

Although parents and media focus on the risk to other children from contact with an HIV-infected child, the primary risk is to the young child with HIV infection. There is no documented case of a teacher, day-care provider, or uninfected child contracting HIV from a child who is HIV positive or who has AIDS.

What can be done to help families who do not have access to supportive, effective social resources? Many of the reservations about providing help are due to misinformation about family needs and misunderstanding about HIV infection. Educating family members and significant others in the family's social network (eg, siblings, grandparents, friends, neighbors, coworkers, teachers, and schoolmates) can deter inappropriate responses that are intended to be supportive and can reduce the social stigma associated with HIV. Mental health or medical professionals can work with families to help them educate those in their social network. Professionals can call "network meetings" to answer questions, share information, and participate in group problem solving, all of which can reduce caregiver stress. In addition, professionals can assist both persons with HIV and family members in the disclosure and grieving process. Although some family members may feel prepared for the death of the child, others may not comprehend the full impact of the loss until after the child has died. Involvement in bereavement groups and hospice work can also be enormously helpful to these families.

The variable most highly related to parenting stress and family functioning in our study was the number of additional caregiving demands made by the child. One way to reduce stress might be to expand the respite care alternatives available to the family. Providing training in special caregiving techniques might be another way to reduce stress. Responding with assistance in the caregiving demands can reduce the stress of daily living tasks that usually are neglected. For example, something as simple as soliciting help with household tasks from family members and friends who have the time and resources to help may greatly alleviate the stress experienced by caregivers. In addition, acquiring the resources and support to assist with the financial strain often reduces a burden that mounts when a caregiver can no longer work or must reduce work hours. Access to entitlement programs should be based on need rather than income so that additional or unusual financial pressures do not deplete personal resources, support, and time.

Emotional support can be sought from other parents of children with HIV infection by joining support groups or just by talking during clinic visits or while in the hospital with the child. Support groups are an important support resource to caregivers coping with HIV infection. Although this study did not allow us to fully examine the support function of support groups, previous investigations[22,23] have found that self-help organizations provide a unique and valuable opportunity for parents feeling alone and overwhelmed to discuss their concerns and fears with other parents of chronically ill children. Some parents in support groups are struggling with the same adjustment problems, while others have experienced the illness situation for a longer period of time and have survived the seemingly insurmountable difficulties of living with HIV. Thus, parents can exchange experienced-based advice and help one another with problem solving. The shared experience of this peer group may serve to affirm the parenting experience of parents coping with HIV infection better than any other sympathetic listener. Caregivers who attended the one support group available at one of the HIV treatment hospitals felt that the support and information gained were very valuable.

Despite the fact that our findings indicate that family functioning is multiply determined, a common thread cut across the fabric of the variables found to be associated with parenting stress and family functioning. As noted earlier, the type and delivery of services needed varied among families, resulting in fragmented services and serious gaps in delivery of services. This suggests that service providers and professionals should be aware that families caring for HIV-infected children have unique individual differences. Because considerable variability was observed among families in their response to alleviating stress and family impact, the need for an Individualized Family Service Plan as called for in Public Law 99-457 is clearly warranted. The presence of HIV infection in a young child should lead these families to early intervention services. Family assessment should include caregivers' perspectives on variables included in the family adaptational model so that services will be aligned with the individual needs and strengths of families.

Several researchers[24,25] have advocated a case management model for coordinating services for families with HIV-infected children. This model can be an effective tool in facilitating appropriate medical treatment and providing coordination for a comprehensive plan of care. However, the efforts of a case manager are often not enough or are not in the best interest to meet the multiple needs of children with HIV infection and their families. One parent succinctly described his experience with case managers by saying, "Case management. Everybody wants to be your case manager but nobody wants to do anything for you." This frustration led some families to not want case managers to coordinate services for them, because they felt that case managers did not listen to their concerns and needs. Some of the families believed that some of the medical and service providers had their own "private agenda." Thus, the efforts of a case manager to support families with HIV-infected children must be done collaboratively through ongoing communication with the family and service providers.

Finally, training to increase staff understanding of HIV infection and its implications for service delivery, flexibility in program implementation, discussion of confidentiality and "right-to-know" issues, and coordination among community agencies are needed to help service providers serve children with HIV infection and their families. Children with HIV infection are clearly in need of developmental and educational supports. Innovative models of service delivery options that are responsive to the changing needs of children and their families need to be developed for this population.

In summary, the findings of our research and of other research in early intervention and pediatric HIV/AIDS programs can inform service providers and can contribute to the development of family and community interventions in the following seven ways:

1. Children and families need early and intense intervention to identify resources within and outside the family that will help them combat their sense of helplessness.
2. An assessment of each family's strengths, needs, and support resources is essential prior to involving the family in an intervention.
3. Most HIV-affected families need assistance with a variety of health, social, educational, and financial problems. Access to such services should be comprehensive and should be done cooperatively with existing social service agencies and community-based service organizations. Differences in families' country of origin, cultural mores, language, religion, and social expectations should be taken into account.
4. Child care for HIV-infected children should be made available. Educational training and basic information about pediatric HIV infection should be provided to all child-care providers to ensure the accessibility and availability of these programs.
5. Innovative solutions will be required to meet the needs of HIV-infected families. Programs should be prepared to provide individualized services to families based on an individualized family assessment. Services should be child centered and family focused. Staff should be trained to understand and be able to respond to families' anxieties and grief.[26]
6. An informal parent and sibling support system should be developed that does not focus solely on the disease, but is a way for families to gain information about resources and referrals and provides an opportunity to share experiences. Preference for meeting times should be parent driven; transportation and child care should be made available.
7. A comprehensive early intervention or school-based developmental program combining such services as regular and special education, physical

therapy, speech therapy, occupational therapy, homebound tutoring, counseling, behavior management, and social work is recommended for all children with HIV infection.[27]

• • •

Research, practice, and policy development relating to HIV-infected children and their families must reflect support for optimal development of these children and families and must address their complex needs. Thus we should give these children and their parents priority status, integrate the information from multiple disciplines into a larger field of endeavor, and then share this information with others. A child's development relies on the coordination and collaboration of social, educational, and medical strategies that will ensure the healthy and orderly development of that child. The challenge for researchers and practitioners becomes one of learning how to better assist HIV-infected children and their families in identifying services that will prevent and remediate this social tragedy.

REFERENCES

1. Simonds RJ, Rogers MF. Epidemiology of HIV in children and other populations. In: Crocker AC, Cohen HJ, Kastner TA, eds. *HIV Infection and Developmental Disabilities.* Baltimore, Md: Brookes Publishing; 1992.
2. Belman AL, Diamond G, Dickson D, et al. Pediatric acquired immunodeficiency syndrome. *Am J Dis Child.* 1988;142:29–35.
3. Epstein LG, Sharer LR, Oleske JM, et al. Neurologic manifestations of human immunodeficiency virus infection in children. *Pediatrics.* 1986;78:678–683.
4. Pizzo PA, Wilfert CM. Treatment considerations for children with human immunodeficiency virus infection. *Pediatr Infect Dis J.* 1990;9:690–699.
5. Plante MC. Caring for the AIDS patient. In: Gong V, Rudnick N, eds. *AIDS: Facts and Issues.* New Brunswick, NJ: Rutgers University Press; 1987.
6. Diamond GW. Developmental problems in children with HIV infection. *Ment Retard.* 1989;27:213–217.
7. Ultmann MH, Belman AL, Ruff HA, et al. Developmental abnormalities in children with acquired immunodeficiency syndrome (AIDS): a follow-up study. *Int J Neurosci.* 1987;32:661–667.
8. Klug R. Children with AIDS. *Am J Nurs.* 1986;86: 1,126–1,132.
9. Bronfenbrenner U. Toward an experimental ecology of human development. *Am Psychol.* 1977;32:513–531.
10. Caplan G. The family as a support system. In: Caplan G, Kililea M, eds. *Support Systems and Mutual Help.* New York, NY: Grune & Stratton; 1976.
11. Cochran M, Brassard J. Child development and personal social networks. *Child Develop.* 1979;50:601–616.
12. Hobbs N. *The Futures of Children.* San Francisco, Calif: Jossey-Bass; 1975.

13. Holahan CJ. Social ecology. In: Iscoe I, Bloom B, Spielberger C, eds. *Community Psychology in Transition.* New York, NY: Wiley; 1977.
14. Mitchell RE, Trickett EJ. Task force report: social networks as mediators of social support. *Community Ment Health J.* 1980;16:27–43.
15. Bronfenbrenner U. *The Ecology of Human Development.* Cambridge, Mass: Harvard University Press; 1979.
16. McCubbin H, Patterson J. The family stress process: the Double ABCX model of adjustment and adaptation. In: McCubbin H, Thompson A, eds. *Social Stress and the Family: Advances and Developments in Family Stress Theory and Research.* New York, NY: Haworth Press; 1983.
17. Dunst CJ, Trivette CM, Deal AG. *Enabling and Empowering Families: Principles and Guidelines for Practice.* Cambridge, Mass: Brookline Books; 1988.
18. Dunst CJ, Jenkins V, Trivette CM. Family support scale: reliability and validity. *J Individ Family Community Wellness.* 1984;1:45–52.
19. McCubbin HI, McCubbin MA, Patterson JM, et al. CHIP—Coping health inventory for parents: an assessment of parental coping patterns in the care of the chronically ill child. *J Marriage Family.* 1983;45:359–370.
20. Stein RE, Riessman CK. The development of an Impact on Family Scale: preliminary findings. *Med Care.* 1980;18:465–472.
21. Friedrich WN, Greenberg MT, Crnic K. A short-form of the questionnaire on resources and stress. *Am J Ment Defic.* 1983;88:41–48.
22. Chesler M, Lebo-Stein J, Barbarin O. Pattern of participation in a self-help group for parents of children with cancer. *J Psychosoc Oncology.* 1984;Fall:49–65.
23. Gussow Z, Tracy GS. The role of self-help clubs in adaptation to chronic illness and disability. *Soc Sci Med.* 1976;10:407–414.
24. Crocker A, Cohen H. *Guidelines on Developmental Services for Children and Adults with HIV Infection.* Silver Spring, Md: American Association of University Affiliated Programs; 1990.
25. Woodruff G, Driscoll P, Sterzin ED. Providing comprehensive and coordinated services to children with HIV infection and their families. In: Crocker A, Cohen TA, eds. *HIV Infection and Developmental Disabilities.* Baltimore, Md: Paul H. Brookes; 1992.
26. Allbritten DJ. *Children with HIV/AIDS: A Sourcebook for Caring.* Alexandria, Va: Stone Webb Print Communication; 1990.
27. Seidel JF. Children with HIV-related developmental difficulties. *Phi Delta Kappan.* 1992;74:38–40.

Early intervention with parents with mental retardation: Do we empower or impair?

Marilyn Espe-Sherwindt, MA
Director, Project CAPABLE
Special Education Department

Sandra L. Kerlin, MEd
Adult Services Consultant
Project CAPABLE
Outreach Continuing Education Department
University Affiliated Cincinnati Center for Developmental Disorders
Cincinnati, Ohio

THE CONCEPT OF empowerment has become a pivotal construct in the planning and implementation of early intervention services for young children (0-2 years) and their families. Implicit in this construct are three frameworks:

1. a proactive framework based on the assumption that parents are competent or are capable of becoming competent;
2. an enabling framework that focuses on creating opportunities for parents to exhibit competence; and
3. an empowering framework that creates opportunities for meeting needs in ways that promote parents' sense of control over their lives and those of their young children.[1]

The notion of empowerment may create conflicts for early intervention professionals faced with parents who at first glance may not seem competent or even capable of becoming competent, that is, parents with mental retardation (MR). Nevertheless, this philosophical perspective is equally valid in delivering services to parents with MR as to any other parent.

UNDERSTANDING PARENTS WITH MENTAL RETARDATION

In many ways, early intervention practitioners are pioneers in working with parents with MR, because, at this time, they have only a partial understanding of how competent parents with MR can be. This dilemma stems from several facts:

This project is supported by Grant #HO24E80020 from the Handicapped Children's Early Education Program, US Department of Education. The development of the pilot early intervention model at UACCDD for parents with special needs was supported by Grant #MCJ 393293, a Special Project of Regional and National Significance (SPRANS), Division of Maternal and Child Health (MCH), US Department of Health and Human Services (DHHS) (7/01/83-6/30/86), and is presently supported by local tax funds. Additional support was provided by Grant #MCJ 000-912-23-0 from the Bureau of Health Care Delivery and Assistance, MCH, DHHS, and Grant #07DD0269/07 from the Administration on Developmental Disabilities, Office of Human Development Services (OHDS), DHHS. The authors acknowledge the assistance of Jack H. Rubinstein, MD, Dorothyann Feldis, PhD, R.J. Gallagher, PhD, Sheila Dove Jones, PhD, and Alexander J. Tymchuk, PhD.

Inf Young Children 1990; 2(4): 21–28

- Such parents have not yet lived in the community with adequate support for a generation.
- Much of the research has included only parents who have been referred by the court for reasons of abuse and/or neglect.
- Studies generally have failed to separate the effects of MR from the effects of living in poverty.[2]

One of the few studies that actually compares the effects of MR with those of poverty used situations that placed the children at risk to compare the decision-making abilities of mothers with MR with those of a control group of mothers with normal intelligence from the same socioeconomic status; no significant differences between the two groups were found.[3] Furthermore, a small but growing body of literature indicates that parents with MR can exhibit increasing competence in certain aspects of parenting. One study[4] used procedures such as discussion, modeling, feedback, and reinforcement to increase the skills of parents with MR in praising appropriate child behaviors and imitating their child's vocalizations; this study demonstrated changes in the parents' behaviors that generalized to the families' home settings and were generally maintained over a follow-up period of 5 to 10 months. In other studies, mothers with MR not only demonstrated gains in the empathy and warmth they provided to their children,[5] but they also learned a deliberative decision-making process, showed increases in the appropriateness of their decisions, and maintained gains in each of these areas during a situational follow-up.[6]

Although there is no direct correlation between higher IQ and parenting ability, certain factors do seem to be helpful in predicting those parents with MR who can provide adequate care for their young children[2]:

- an IQ greater than 50,
- being married,
- having fewer children,
- adequate financial support, and
- adequate, accepted support from formal and informal sources.

The parallels between these factors and those protective factors identified by the 30-year Kauai Longitudinal Project[7] of high-risk infants as promoting positive outcomes are striking: what emerges is a pattern of support for parents with or without MR, from sources ranging from spouse to family to friends to professionals to community.

Successful early intervention for parents with MR may require an initial, but crucial preliminary step, what Turnbull and Turnbull[8] described as "empathetic reciprocity." "This principle requires us to put ourselves in the place of others as fully as we can, looking at the world from their perspectives and using their values and needs. It requires us to do something very hard: to put our own perspectives, values, and needs on the shelf."[8(p106)] Such empathy can be especially difficult for professionals working with these parents, since early interventionists may have had little experience with adults with MR that could truly be described as "life-sharing." Instead, owing to the historic segregation of people with special needs or MR, professionals may be influenced by stereotypes (eg, that persons with mental retardation are either aggressive and dangerous or loving and childlike), rather than personal experience. The behaviors of parents with MR may be misconstrued as hostile, disinterested, and neglectful, when in reality these parents are reacting to a lifelong learning experience of being regarded as incapable, "second-class" citizens. Consequently, professionals unintentionally may equate MR with parental incompetence.

To understand the behaviors of parents with special needs or MR, it is helpful to consider five areas of functioning: (1) internal/external control, (2) self-esteem, (3) social skills, (4) social role comprehension, and (5) problem-solving skills. Consider, for example, that many adults with MR have been taught through external control methods; response, not reasoning, has been the mainstay of many special education programs.[9] Self-direction, internalization of reward, and the value of appropriate human interaction have not necessarily been part of their life experiences.

Many techniques used to control or change behavior, especially of institutionalized individuals, have been punishing rather than rewarding, and, consequently, the rewards of human presence and interaction have not been taught.[10] It is difficult to perform the many and varied routine tasks of parenting if one responds only to external "reward." Parenting in and of itself is often a "giving" task that reaps no immediate tangible reward. The adult with MR who has been excessively controlled or coerced as a child may as an adult passively submit to or rely to an excessive degree on the direction of others, thereby ignoring cues from his or her own child.

It is also possible that ignoring the task at hand, forgetting, procrastinating, and daydreaming will be part of the adult's life style.[11] If we persist in treating adults with MR as children, then their response to parenting is likely to be childlike. Consequently, the concept of empowerment clearly addresses a crucial issue for parents with MR who may need encouragement and skill development to experience the rewards of internal control.

Healthy self-esteem is closely related to social adjustment and to the acceptance of the responsibilities of parenthood. Because segregation and frequent failure (both academic and social) in childhood and adolescence may have been primary to the learning experience of adults with MR, their self-esteem is likely to be damaged. Continued rejection may cause the development of bitter, hostile, and anxious feelings in an adult who is self-depreciating and has severe difficulty relating to and being close to others.[11] The positive recognition of accomplishments is vital to the development of self-esteem. It seems significant that praising the child has been found to be the single maternal behavior most absent in mothers with MR and that this absence of praising is tied to the mothers' low self-esteem.[4,5,12] Building parental self-esteem cannot be overlooked in providing early intervention services to parents with MR.

Social skills are equally important to the task of parenting. Parents who know how to obtain services, talk to professionals, and ask the right questions are considered to be interested, adequate parents. The social skills of adults with MR may be limited in scope, because most social skills are learned through social interaction and contact. As expectations for people with MR have been very limited by society, even those individuals growing up in nurturing families may have been socially isolated. Adults with MR have not been taught to seek out needed services and for the most part have no experience in voluntarily consulting with "professionals": they have been "taken to" services or had services brought to them. Training in the use of the community and in social interaction is vital to the development of social skills that will enable the parent with MR to obtain what is needed for himself or herself and the child. For example, a mother in an early intervention program indicates that she wants books for her children. Instead of buying books for her or giving or lending books to her, the interventionist should develop an alternative strategy. If this mother is shown how to reach the public library, how to acquire a library card, how to check out and return books, and how to interact with the library staff, she is empowered to gain for her children and herself what she determines is needed.

Being able to take on various social roles as an adult often depends on defined expectations and on having a clear understanding of the experience with those roles. For the adult with MR, the roles of independent adult and parent are likely to be very new. Persons who learn to be adequate parents have primarily learned those skills from their parents. Children are taught good parenting in a very natural way because it is expected that they may someday be parents, too; if that is not the expectation, not much attention will be paid to the task. For the most part, regardless of where adults with MR have grown up (loving home or institution), the issues of sexuality, parenting, and social role development have not been addressed.

It is now recognized that "people labelled as mentally retarded are perhaps the last amongst the various client groups to be considered autonomous individuals with a say in their own destinies."[13(p213)] If they are to have a "say," problem-solving skills must be developed. However, although volumes of information exist to teach individuals with disabilities academic and technical skills, there is a "dearth of curricula for teaching students how to pinpoint and define problems, generate and evaluate alternatives, select the preferred alternative, take action, and evaluate the consequences of their action."[9(p116)] It is unrealistic and unfair to expect adults with MR to solve the multiple problems related to adequate parenting without recognizing and redressing the situation that they were *not taught* problem-solving skills as children and adolescents. As parenting is now a reality for adults with

MR, the teaching of problem solving must also become real. The remainder of this article will explore the relationship between an understanding of parents with MR and the development of empowering early intervention services.

LINKING KNOWLEDGE WITH INTERVENTION

A philosophical framework

In 1983, the University Affiliated Cincinnati Center for Developmental Disorders (UACCDD) received funding through a 3-year grant from the Maternal and Child Health Special Projects of Regional and National Significance (SPRANS) to develop a model early intervention program for infants with or at risk for developmental disabilities born to high-risk parents who were unable to use existing early intervention resources for reasons related both to the family and to the service delivery system. The primary objectives of the project were

1. to establish a trusting partnership between families and staff;
2. to enable families, through increased self-esteem, social skills, and problem-solving skills, to obtain improved parent–child interactions;
3. to enable families to understand that their experiences with professionals and the service delivery system can be rewarding rather than punitive;
4. to build a collaborative network of support and services, in the realization that no one agency has the staff or financial resources to meet all needs of all families; and
5. to support the successful transition of families to community-based services, with the recognition that these families may need to access a long-term support system.

Now in its sixth year, the UACCDD program has served 39 children in 30 families in which one or both parents have been identified as having MR on the basis of information provided by the family or referring agency. The average age of children at entry into the program was 11.3 months. The parents were married in 13 of the 30 families. The mean length of stay in the program for these families was 34.6 weeks. Follow-up data indicate that of these 30 families, 17 (22 children) are currently intact and are involved in services (eg, Head Start program or being monitored by public health or social service agencies); five families have had their children (7) placed in temporary foster care but are working toward reunification. Eight children in six families have been permanently removed. Only two families have been lost to follow-up.

The commonalities that emerged among the families who have remained together are consistent with the literature citing social support as a significant protective factor. These families had several key figures (both family members and professionals) who believed in their ability and who provided opportunities for competence to emerge. Those families whose children were removed permanently were characterized by a limited support system, the loss of a key support figure at a crucial time, or the continued view of them by key figures as incompetent.

Strategies for intervention

Early intervention for families in which parents have MR does not occur quickly or easily. The UACCDD experience indicates that establishing a trusting relationship with parents with MR is the key first step in providing effective early intervention. The concept of partnership implicit in Public Law 99-457, that is, a shared responsibility with the professional serving in a facilitator role, is as important for the parent with MR as for all other parents. This partnership may prove to be a lengthy process, but it can be facilitated through focusing on the needs most crucial to the parent, being nonjudgmental and affirming, and "nurturing" or "reparenting" the parent while providing concrete assistance. The experiences of the UACCDD program also support the assertion that intervention for these families "needs to begin with the problem of social support."[14(p1154)] Parenting and child development per se cannot be a priority as long as families are overwhelmed by the crises of day-to-day survival. Bromwich[15] stressed the need to begin intervention with a dual focus: (1) identifying areas of most critical stress for the family and supporting the family in alleviating those concerns, while (2) ensuring that the basic survival needs of the infant are being met. Once a trusting relationship has been established and the most immediate survival crises have been at least partially resolved, intervention priorities can be shifted toward parenting and child development issues. This perspective may prove to be frustrating to professionals in early intervention, particularly if their training has been child-focused rather than family-focused. They may feel that their own skills are being wasted or underused, and thus will resent the time and effort needed to provide social support and crisis intervention to these families—especially as it often reaps minimal immediate results.

It is important to keep in mind the intent of Public Law 99-457, that "intervention efforts should be based on family-identified needs and aspirations in order to have the greatest positive influences on child, parent, and family functioning."[16(p34)] Parents with MR can—within the context of a safe, trusting, enabling relationship—identify priorities for themselves and their children. For example, a mother and her 10-month-old son were referred to the UACCDD program by her protective caseworker, who was concerned about the mother's abilities to marshal her resources and interact with her child. It quickly became apparent that the mother perceived the early intervention services to be intrusive and potentially punitive, and that she masked this fear by reiterating that she was an adequate mother who had no needs for information, support, or services.

The program staff was faced with several options: (1) to label the mother as resistant and terminate services; (2) to "clarify" for her what her needs were and how the program could help; or (3) to look for, acknowledge, and encourage strengths in the mother and "wait for the door to open." On a home visit several weeks later, it was evident that there were no toys available for the infant; the mother explained that the toys had been stolen. This exchange was used by the mother to clarify her desire for toys for her infant, a need that was important to her and that she felt she could do something about. Several responses by the staff were possible: (1) give her toys; (2) take her to a toy store and help her choose "developmentally appropriate" toys; or (3) provide opportunities for the mother to make toys that would not only build her self-esteem, but also promote interactions between her and her child. This last option was consistent with the concept of empowerment, and during the next several sessions of the program, the mother chose one of several options for making toys, talked enthusiastically with the staff while she was working, and commented on how much her infant would enjoy playing with the toy she was making. This mother subsequently has attended the program regularly, has demonstrated increasing interactions with both the staff and her child, and has entered an alcoholism treatment program.

Various curricula and resources are available to assist early intervention professionals in addressing the priorities in the areas of child development and parenting that are identified *together with* parents with MR.[17–20] A familiarity with such resources along with knowledge of adult learning theory,[21] an understanding of nonverbal teaching techniques, and the use of repetition, rehearsal, and feedback are important strategies in working with parents with MR. However, because no one curriculum magically fits all families, success in the use of such resources and strategies depends strongly on the relationship established between parent and professional. If program personnel intend to provide families with appropriate services, as determined by each family's priorities and unique functioning, then intervention must be tailor-made to each parent with MR.

An overemphasis on curricula may obscure the key principles of enabling and empowering. Early intervention professionals may lament the inability of parents with MR to generalize skills and to anticipate developmental changes in their children; they may need to reconsider that they have been promoting discrete skills rather than developing generic, underlying processes. Early intervention programs may unintentionally continue the lifelong experiences of these persons of someone identifying for them a "functional skill" and teaching a series of responses; what emerges is a passive person who continues to wait for an external cue. Although it is very important to provide opportunities for these parents to learn skills (rather than teaching them) such as diapering, bathing, making formula, and promoting their child's development, the UACCDD program has found that it is helpful to pursue experience in other areas that not only are more "generalizable," but also promote self-esteem, internal control, and competence.

Incorporation of the concepts of decision making,[6] as well as a focus on responsive, child-oriented style of parent–child interaction and turn taking,[22] encourages in these parents an increased competence in underlying processes that has long-term implications. One study of mothers with MR[23] reported a stronger positive correlation between the quality of maternal–child interactions and the child's cognitive development at age 2 than between maternal IQ and developmental outcome. Early interventionists should not overlook themselves as a catalyst for change; positive interaction between the professional and the parent with MR can become a means of promoting self-esteem, social skills, problem solving—that is, empowerment.[24]

Evaluating progress

Change, which can be both slow and seemingly minute, is a major source of frustration to professionals working with parents with MR. The method called Goal Attainment Scaling,[25] used in conjunction with goals developed as part of the Individualized Family Service Plan, presents itself as a valuable evaluation tool, because it requires programs to categorize the expectations for individual families from the worst to the best outcome.[25,26] Given the fact that traditional methods of measuring change (eg, paper and pencil tests, detailed observational measures) may not be optimal for these families or for service providers, it is crucial to view change in alternative, even unlikely ways, such as excellent program attendance by a family previously viewed by multiple agencies as an uncooperative "no-show." One survey indicated that a positive outcome of training with parents with MR was associated with the degree to which the mothers were involved in treatment.[27]

Another source of documented change can be found in extensive clinical notes and case studies reporting both progress at the program site, such as increasing interactions with child and staff, and feedback from other agencies or family members, such as the report from a homemaker sent into the home by the Department of Human Services that the mother is following through in her interactions with the child using the activities reinforced during the early intervention program. Increased successful problem solving by these families, documented similarly, suggests that they are beginning to generalize new skills acquired through intervention. Such data collection can be planned systematically to match the objectives of the program. Another nontraditional indicator of success may be a family's ability to stay "in the system," which suggests that the family has come to view professionals as trustworthy resources, that the needs of their child have become a priority, and that the family has begun to acquire the requisite skills for successful navigation within the service delivery system.

Linking intervention with training

Training in early intervention traditionally has not provided the skills needed to work effectively with parents with MR. Clearly, these skills can be identified[28] and should be incorporated into preservice programs as they are developed by institutions of higher education. The inservice education needs of early interventionists in the field are similar, but have also not been addressed. Project CAPABLE (**C**ommunities **A**ssisting **P**arents to be **ABLE**), an early intervention outreach project at UACCDD, is providing inservice training, ongoing technical assistance, and development of materials for personnel in programs serving (or interested in serving) children from birth through 2 years at established, biologic, or environmental risk who have parents with MR. Because a positive relationship between the professional and parent is the most valuable curriculum resource for effecting change with parents with MR, both preservice and inservice training must focus not only on knowledge and skills, but also on the values and attitudes that professionals hold toward these families. Consequently, CAPABLE has developed a training approach that incorporates these components.

• • •

Parents with MR may indeed have difficulty solving "the ever-changing problems that must be confronted as their children grow and develop."[29(p33)] Most parents do at one time or other. However, if these same parents can be provided with the social and problem-solving skills that enable them to identify their own periodic needs for assistance, to view asking for help as enabling rather than disabling, and to access the appropriate support systems—and if early interventionists can develop through preservice and inservice training the skills necessary to establish partnerships with parents with MR—then empowerment will have occurred for the families who most need our assistance.

REFERENCES

1. Dunst CJ, Trivette CM, Deal AG. *Enabling and Empowering Families: Principles and Guidelines for Practice.* Cambridge, Mass: Brookline Books; 1988.
2. Tymchuk AJ, Andron L, Unger O. Parents with mental handicaps and adequate child care—a review. *Ment Handicap.* 1987;15:49–54.
3. Tymchuk AJ, Yokota A, Rahbar B. Decision-making abilities of mothers with mental retardation. Unpublished manuscript, 1988.
4. Feldman MA, Towns F, Betel J, et al. Parent Education Project II: increasing stimulating interactions of developmentally handicapped mothers. *J Appl Behav Anal.* 1986;19:23–37.
5. Tymchuk AJ, Andron L. Clinic and home parent training of a mother with mental handicap caring for three children with developmental delay. *Ment Handicap Res.* 1988;1(1):24–38.
6. Tymchuk AJ, Andron L, Rahbar B. Effective decision-making/problem-solving training with mothers who have mental retardation. *Am J Ment Retard.* 1988;92(6):510–516.
7. Werner EE. Individual differences, universal needs: 30-year study of resilient high risk infants. *Zero to Three.* National Center for Clinical Infant Programs, Washington, DC, 1988;8:1–5.
8. Turnbull AP, Turnbull HR. Stepping back from early intervention: an ethical perspective. *J Div Early Child.* 1986;10(2):106–117.

9. Turnbull AP, Turnbull HR. Developing independence. *J Adolesc Health Care.* 1985;6:108–119.
10. McGee W, Menolascino F, Hobbs DC, et al. *Gentle Teaching: A Nonaversive Approach for Helping Persons with Mental Retardation.* New York: Human Sciences Press; 1987.
11. Marlin K. *Practical Parenting: Parenting Styles That Handicap Children.* Columbia, Mo: Practical Parenting Publications; 1976.
12. Peterson SL, Robinson EA, Littman I. Parent–child interaction training for parents with a history of mental retardation. *Appl Res Ment Retard.* 1983;4:329–342.
13. Brechin A, Swain J. Professional/client relationships: creating a "working alliance" with people with learning difficulties. *Disability, Handicap & Society.* 1988;3(3):213–226.
14. Bee HL, Barnard KE, Eyres SJ, et al. Prediction of IQ and language skill from perinatal status, child performance, family characteristics and mother–infant interaction. *Child Dev.* 1982;53:1134–1156.
15. Bromwich R. "Vulnerable infants" and "risky environments." *Zero to Three.* National Center for Clinical Infant Programs, Washington, DC, 1985;6:7–12.
16. Deal AG, Dunst CJ, Trivette CM. A flexible and functional approach to developing Individualized Family Support Plans. *Inf Young Children.* 1989;1(4):32–43.
17. Graves B, Graves D, Haynes Y, et al. *Parents Learning Together: A Curriculum for Use with MR/DD Parents.* St. Louis: St. Louis Office for Mental Retardation/Developmental Disabilities Resources; 1986.
18. Parks S. *HELP: When the Parent Is Handicapped.* Palo Alto: VORT Corporation; 1984.
19. Andron L, Deacon S. *Parenting Birth to SW: For Parents with Special Learning Needs.* Los Angeles: American Red Cross, Los Angeles Chapter; 1988.
20. Espe-Sherwindt M, Kerlin SL. Project CAPABLE. *I Love Somebody: Safety in the Home* (videotape and discussion leader's manual). Cincinnati: University Affiliated Cincinnati Center for Developmental Disorders; 1989.
21. Sakata RT. *Adult Education: Theory and Practice.* Chapel Hill, NC: Technical Assistance Development System; 1984.
22. Mahoney G, Powell A. Modifying parent–child interaction: enhancing the development of handicapped children. *J Spec Educ.* 1988;22:82–96.
23. Feldman MA, Case L, Towns F, et al. Parent Education Project I: development and nurturance of children of mentally retarded parents. *Am J Ment Defic.* 1985;90(3):255–258.
24. Booth CL, Mitchell SK, Barnard KE, et al. Development of maternal social skills in multiproblem families: effects on the mother–child relationship. *Dev Psychol.* 1989;25:403–412.
25. Bailey DB. Considerations in developing family goals. In: Bailey DB, Simeonsson RJ, eds. *Family Assessment in Early Intervention.* Columbus, Ohio: Merrill Publishing; 1988.
26. Simeonsson RJ. Evaluating the effects of family-focused intervention. In: Bailey DB, Simeonsson RJ, eds. *Family Assessment in Early Intervention.* Columbus, Ohio: Merrill Publishing; 1988.
27. Budd KS, Greenspan S. Parameters of successful and unsuccessful interventions with parents who are mentally retarded. *Ment Retard.* 1985;23(6):269–273.
28. Espe-Sherwindt M, Kerlin SL. Skills for partnerships with parents with special needs/mental retardation. In: Espe-Sherwindt M, Beatty CL, eds. *New Perspectives on Partnering with Families: Implications for Training Early Intervention Personnel (Selected Proceedings).* Cincinnati: University Affiliated Cincinnati Center for Developmental Disorders; 1989.
29. Lynch EW, Bakley S. Serving young children whose parents are mentally retarded. *Inf Young Children.* 1989;1(3):26–38.

Adolescent mothers and their premature infants: Responding to double risk

S. Kenneth Thurman, PhD
Professor of Special Education
Department of Psychological Studies
in Education
Temple University
Philadelphia, Pennsylvania

Sonia V. Gonsalves, PhD
Assistant Professor of Psychology
Department of Behavioral Sciences
Stockton State College
Pomona, New Jersey

KOPP (1987) has asserted that "the phrase *developmental risk* indicates the well-being of children is in jeopardy."[1(p881)] The degree of risk to an individual child is determined by both biologic and environmental factors. Biologic risk is due to factors such as prematurity, genetic disorders, respiratory distress, and prenatal drug exposure. Environmental risk includes factors such as poverty, lack of nurturance, and nonsynchronous interaction between child and caregiver. A decade and a half ago Parmelee et al[2,3] and Sameroff and Chandler[4] first suggested that environmental and biologic risk factors combine to determine the actual risk status of an infant or young child. Parmelee et al[2,3] suggest that these factors combine into what they termed cumulative risk. The cumulative risk index provides an indication of the likelihood of developmental outcomes that are less than optimal. Similarly, Field et al suggested that "being born both preterm and to a teenage mother appears to place the infant at greater risk than simply being born preterm or to a teenage mother."[5(p434)] This article discusses how prematurity and single teenage motherhood combine to create a cumulative or double risk for infants. In addition, we describe the factors that are unique to these mothers and their children and the components of a service delivery model designed to be responsive to their needs.

SPECIFIC CONDITIONS CONTRIBUTING TO DOUBLE RISK

The premature birth of an infant and the hospitalization that follows can be a time of intense feelings for an adolescent mother with little experience in parenthood. She may feel depressed, happy, angry, scared, guilty, competent, and incompetent, in combination or independently. Clearly these intense and often conflicting feelings can affect the manner in which the young mother interacts with her infant. How this young mother relates to and interacts with her infant during the neonatal period and beyond sets in motion a series of transactions that will help determine the course of her infant's development.[4]

The literature documents that adolescent mothers, compared with their more mature counterparts, may be less verbal in interacting with their infants,[6,7] may be less adept at reading their infants' cues,[7] and may respond to their infants in less contingent ways.[8] In addition, adolescent mothers may exhibit less knowledge

Inf Young Children 1993; 5(4): 44–51

about child development[9–11] and a greater tendency toward child abuse compared with older mothers.[9,10]

The fact that the earliest interactions between adolescent mothers and their preterm infants take place in a neonatal intensive care unit (NICU) can further affect responding.[12] These young mothers must contend with the apparently chaotic nature and lack of privacy often associated with the NICU. Lawson et al[13] a number of years ago recognized that NICUs are bright and noisy and expose infants to large amounts of nonsocial stimuli, which others have noted are often not delivered to the infants in a contingent manner.[14] These factors too may interfere with the young mother's interactions with her infant.

Early visits even by more mature mothers to the NICU have been characterized as tenuous.[15,16] Furthermore, Minde et al[17] have reported that during early visits to the NICU mothers may be less confident and more passive, preferring to look at their infants rather than to interact more actively with them. They also reported that with the passage of time mothers become more actively involved with their infants. Minde et al[15] have also presented data that suggest that mothers who are more active in the NICU are also more actively involved with their infants during the first 3 months at home.

Even after the infant is discharged from the hospital, differences in patterns of interaction persist. Mothers of premature or ill infants may respond differently to their children than mothers of full-term, healthy infants. Mothers of preterm infants may be less actively involved, may make less body contact,[18] may spend less time in face-to-face contact,[19] and may smile at, touch, and talk to their infants less.[20,21] In addition, Greene et al[22] have reported that mothers show less affective expression to their preterm infants at 3 months. This result is in contrast to findings by Crawford,[23] who reported that mothers of these infants show more affectionate responses to their infants. In another study, mothers and their premature infants were less able to coordinate their cycles of affective behavior during social interaction.[24] The more ambiguous cues provided by preterm infants lead to increased maternal efforts to engage the infant, which in turn lead to the infant's averting its gaze and thus shutting down the interaction.[25,26] As a result these patterns of interaction are often much less synchronous and reciprocal than those of mothers with their healthy full-term babies.

Many characteristics of preterm infants put them at risk for developing less than optimal patterns of social interactions with their caregivers. Behaviorally, these infants are less active, initiate fewer interactions, and provide less feedback to their caregivers than their full-term peers.[20,27] Furthermore, these infants maintain less eye contact with their mothers, avert their gaze more, smile less,[21,28] use more unclear signals,[25,29] and are more difficult to cuddle and console than their term peers.[22]

Additional risk factors accrue because of the adolescent status of the mother. Children of adolescent mothers are more likely to be born into and to continue to live in poverty and to be physically, emotionally, and intellectually compromised as they develop.[30] The adolescent mother herself has educational and economic disadvantages. These young women are less likely to complete high school and are more likely to have larger families and to continue to live in poverty. Prater[31] suggests that many of these young women were doing poorly in school when they became pregnant. Giving birth and taking on the demands of motherhood usually decrease their school performance further and often are precipitating factors in their decision to drop out.

In summary, it is clear that various factors combine to put infants at risk when they are born prematurely and when their mothers are adolescents. These factors lead to some specific concerns that must be recognized if interventions are to be put into place that will help reduce the risk to these infants and their young mothers.

SPECIFIC CONCERNS FOR PRETERM INFANTS AND THEIR ADOLESCENT MOTHERS

Adolescent mothers and their preterm infants may fail to become attached because of the separation resulting from the infant's protracted hospital stay, the infant's inability to engage the mother for the first several weeks of life, fear on the part of the mother of becoming attached to an infant who appears to have a tenuous hold on life, and the lack of a clear parenting role for the mother during the infant's hospitalization. In addition, the first-time young mother may be uncertain about her skills as a parent. Often, too, it may be difficult for her to get to the hospital because of lack of transportation. Without some early intervention aimed at supporting the relationship between the mother and infant, there is every likelihood that the relationship will suffer. Such support should start within the first few days of the infant's hospitalization, while the mother is still in the hospital recovering from delivery. This intervention must stay in place throughout the infant's hospitalization if it is to be maximally beneficial.

The adolescent mother must be made to feel comfortable in the NICU. The NICU environment can be intimidating to an adolescent. The monitors, ventilators, and alarms, the lack of privacy, the preponderance of authority figures, and the infant's fragile condition all militate against an adolescent mother's willingness to visit the NICU and to spend time with her infant. These young women need support in overcoming their anxiety and fear regarding the NICU. If a mother remains afraid of the NICU setting, she is not likely to be inclined to visit her infant.

Besides her fear and anxiety, a young mother may not have appropriate social skills to take the best advantage of the NICU environment. Adolescents tend to be excessively self-conscious. This self-consciousness is characterized by the feeling that the world is noticing and judging every move that the adolescent makes. Elkind[32,33] and Elkind and Bowen[34] have termed this feeling of transparency the imaginary audience. Adolescent mothers tend to be hypersensitive about their behavior, and their self-confidence is disproportionately affected by the slightest remark that they consider censorial. Physicians and nurses may not be actively regarding the adolescent status of these mothers and may not consider the fragility of their self-esteem. Consequently, they may inadvertently alienate these young women.

Furthermore, the adolescent mother may not display behaviors that medical personnel associate with a concerned parent. These mothers may not ask appropriate questions regarding their infant's course. They may seem unconcerned and preoccupied. Hospital personnel may hold them to standards that are more likely to be met by older and more experienced mothers. Physicians and nurses may hold preconceptions that cause them to react to adolescent mothers differently than they do to older mothers. Adolescent mothers often are sensitive to these subtle differences in the behavior of professionals and will react with alienation and hurt feelings.

Adams and Gulotta[35] have suggested several parameters that, if adhered to, will increase the likelihood of success in working with adolescent mothers: trustworthiness, genuine regard, empathy, and honesty. These investigators suggest that no age group is more adept at detecting phony regard than adolescents. Too often, hospital personnel are unfamiliar with the parameters suggested by Adams and Gulotta,[35] and consequently their success in working with adolescent mothers is inhibited. Thurman et al[36] have stressed the importance of staff development efforts aimed at making NICU staff more aware of issues in working with adolescents, which can lead to young mothers feeling more comfortable in the NICU.

Like other mothers, adolescent mothers may feel guilt in association with the birth of their preterm infant. These feelings may be exacerbated because the young mother is unaware of the causes of prematurity. She may even attribute her infant's situation to events and behaviors during her pregnancy that have no relationship to her infant's prematurity. A mother's feelings of guilt may contribute to her tendency not to visit because confronting her infant will bring forward her guilty feelings. It is important to help adolescent mothers understand their infant's condition while minimizing their feelings of guilt.

Adolescents are accustomed to activity and may have difficulty in the NICU because there are limited opportunities to interact and be involved in activities. The young mother is unable to play with her infant, and early in the course of hospitalization she may not be able to participate in the infant's care. Often she is just sitting and watching her infant. In the absence of a clear role in the NICU, the young mother may see another reason not to visit her infant. She may feel that it makes no difference whether she shows up because her infant does not know she is there and there is nothing for her to do once she arrives. It is often more reinforcing and more comfortable for the young mother to stay away and be in the neighborhood with her friends. Often she is not permitted to bring friends to the NICU and thus is unable to share her experience with them directly. Furthermore, she may be receiving little support from the infant's father. In many cases it is the adolescent's own mother who is a primary source of support and encouragement. Efforts should be made to develop support systems for these young women, whether the support comes from their own mothers, other family or friends, or professionals. Just being permitted to bring a friend along to visit in the NICU may make an adolescent mother feel more comfortable and may reduce her level of stress.

Adolescent mothers are more likely to have exaggerated expectations of their infant. They lack knowledge of child development and thus may attribute abilities to their infants that are unrealistic even for the full-term newborn. Typically, young mothers are not aware of the possibility of premature birth and have limited knowledge of it and its implications. If they are not given explanations about their infant that are clear and understandable to them, they are likely to feel frustrated and inadequate in their role as a mother.

Adolescent mothers, like all adolescents, are seeking identity and autonomy. The birth of their infant further complicates this process. The adolescent mother must seek her identity not only as a person but also as a mother. Her search for autonomy is affected by the responsibilities she now has in caring for her infant.

Adolescents often have difficulty planning for the future. They are oriented toward the gratification available in the present environment. They may see their responsibility for their infant as an impediment to that gratification. This can lead to feelings of resentment toward the infant.

The adolescent mother's difficulty in making and carrying out plans is exacerbated by her relative lack of academic and vocational preparation. As noted previously,[32] the birth of her infant may further limit the likelihood that she will return to school. A consequence of these typical adolescent traits may lead professionals working with them to perceive these young mothers as irresponsible and uncaring. In actuality, it is important for professionals to provide these young women with support and guidance and to create for them opportunities that will enhance their academic, vocational, and planning skills.

PARAMETERS FOR INTERVENTION WITH A DOUBLE-RISK POPULATION

The construct of cumulative risk[2,3] discussed above is fundamental to any intervention designed for this population. The cumulative risk construct recognizes that multiple factors combine to define the risk status of the child and family. It further leads to the recognition that environmental factors are often more easily modifiable than the biologic ones that contribute to the infant's vulnerability.

A second parameter that underlies the development of interventions for this population is the recognition that early maternal–infant interaction provides an important contribution to the eventual developmental outcomes of premature infants. This premise has been supported by Lewis and Goldberg[37] and Sameroff and Chandler,[4] among others. Thus intervention must focus on the relationship between the mother and her infant and on their mutual responding to each other.

A third parameter that is crucial to the development of programs for this population grows from the ecologic perspectives presented by Bronnfenbrenner,[38,39] Thurman,[40,41] and Thurman and Widerstrom.[42] These perspectives suggest that the interaction between the system and the individual is key to the determination of outcome and function. Thus there is a relationship between the improvement of a system and the improvement of the individuals within that system. Furthermore, the degree of fit among the individuals in the system and the degree of fit between the individuals and the physical environment help determine developmental outcomes for individuals.[40–42] Accordingly, interventions should be designed that help develop and maintain the best interactive fit between mothers and their infants. Empowerment of young mothers will contribute to their abilities to facilitate the development of systems with a high degree of fit for themselves and their infants.

THE PAIR PROJECT—AN EXAMPLE OF A MODEL PROGRAM FOR RESPONDING TO DOUBLE RISK

The Parents and Infants Responding (PAIR) Project was funded through the Early Education for Children with Disabilities Program administered by the Office of Special Education, Department of Education.[36] The PAIR Project was responsive to the concerns and parameters discussed above in developing and implementing services for adolescent mothers and their premature infants.

The PAIR Project was based at Temple University Hospital in Philadelphia and provided services to single adolescent mothers and their premature infants beginning with the infant's birth. The main focus of the PAIR Project was developing adaptive fit between mothers and their infants. In addition, the project was designed to provide mothers with social support while leading them to empowered independence. The PAIR Project was staffed by two professionals called parent/infant facilitators, who had the responsibility of implementing PAIR Project services. They were supervised by the project coordinator and could draw on the services of a neonatologist, occupational therapist, physical therapist, and speech/language therapist as needed.

The PAIR Project interventions were based on a four-component model. Each component was designed to contribute to increasing the mother's ability to support herself and her infant. The four components of the PAIR model were engagement, intervention, maintenance, and empowerment. The engagement component focused on the mother's initial interaction with the infant and stressed the development of a partnership between the mothers and the project staff. The intervention component grew from the assessment of mother–infant interactions and each infant's developmental needs. Interventions, such as helping a mother respond more contingently to her infant's cues, were based on these assessments and were implemented by project staff. When possible, mothers and infants were referred to and placed into existing community services. The maintenance component was based on the ongoing partnership between the mother and the staff and focused on putting into place the necessary supports to maintain the optimal interaction between mother and infant and to help ensure the infant's developmental progress. The empowerment component focused on enabling the mothers to take control of their own lives as well as their infants. Mothers were assisted with educational and vocational needs and were aided in establishing goals for themselves and in reaching them independently.

Interventions were begun when each infant was born. Mothers were approached in the hospital, and the project's services were explained to them. They were provided with the names of the staff and were encouraged to visit their infant in the NICU as many times as possible during their own hospital stay. The parent/infant facilitators made home visits to the mothers and helped them get back and forth to visit their infant at the hospital. They provided mothers with suggestions about child care, patterns of interaction, and available community services. A parent/infant facilitator formed a partnership with each mother assigned to her and helped mothers become more empowered and independent over time. They helped mothers prepare for bringing their infant home. PAIR provided various layette items for the infants as needed, and the parent/infant facilitators continued to make home visits, during which they assisted the mothers in setting goals and implementing plans. In addition, they monitored the development of each infant and made suggestions to the mothers regarding activities that they could do with their infant. When necessary, the parent/infant facilitators consulted with appropriate therapists and made referrals to more intensive early intervention programs when an infant's developmental pattern suggested that that was necessary. Mothers were encouraged and supported in their efforts to finish high school or to seek additional vocational training or higher education as appropriate. Monthly group social activities were held, during which mothers were able to support each other and to share experiences. In addition to the social aspects of these gatherings, guest speakers were brought in to provide the mothers with relevant information concerning the development of infants and toddlers or self-improvement opportunities for the young women. The length of time that a mother and her infant continued to receive PAIR services was, like the type and degree of services, individually determined.

Although it is beyond the scope of this article to discuss fully the evaluation of PAIR's effectiveness, we are collecting data to assess the effectiveness of the project. The evaluation is based on the comparison of outcomes of the mothers and infants served by PAIR with outcomes of a contrast group of mothers who received routine hospital services. Initial data suggest that PAIR met its goal of increasing maternal visitation. An initial comparison shows that PAIR mothers visited their infants more proportionately than contrast mothers (0.64 compared to 0.54). Interestingly, the contrast mothers showed a higher proportion of phone calls (0.54 compared to 0.37). A tentative interpretation of these results is that PAIR services were effective in getting mothers to visit their infants rather than depending on phone calls to get information. Contrast infants also had a longer mean length of stay than infants served by PAIR (59.6 days compared to 48.2 days). This difference is not attributable to gestational age, which was essentially identical for PAIR infants (mean, 29.7 weeks) and contrast infants (mean, 29.6 weeks).

Both groups of mothers were also given a measure to determine the personal impact of having an infant in an NICU. Again, initial data suggest that the contrast group mothers experienced a stronger impact than the PAIR mothers. Contrast group mothers had a mean score of 25.75 on this measure; PAIR mothers had a mean score of 18.10. A higher score was indicative of more impact.

Although these data are all initial and are based on partial samples of each group, they are nonetheless, when taken as a whole, suggestive of PAIR's effectiveness. Further data collection to assess PAIR's effectiveness centers on patterns of mother–infant interaction, maternal empowerment, and maternal knowledge of child development. In addition, the developmental status of the infants is being assessed periodically until they reach their third birthdays.

• • •

This article has discussed the factors that contribute to the increased risk to infants who are born prematurely to adolescent mothers. To be successful with this population, it is necessary for interventionists to understand not only infant and toddler development and how it is affected by prematurity but also the development of adolescents and how that development is affected by parenthood.

REFERENCES

1. Kopp CB. Developmental risk: historical reflections. In: Osofsky JD, ed. *Handbook of Infant Development.* New York, NY: Wiley; 1987.
2. Parmelee AH, Sigman M, Kopp CB, Haber A. The concept of a cumulative risk score. In: Ellis NR, ed. *Aberrant Development in Infancy: Human and Animal Studies.* Hillsdale, NJ: Erlbaum; 1975.
3. Parmelee AH, Sigman M, Kopp CB, Haber A. Diagnosis of the infant at high risk for mental, motor, and sensory handicaps. In: Tjossem TD, ed. *Intervention Strategies for High Risk Infants and Young Children.* Baltimore, Md: University Park Press; 1976.
4. Sameroff AJ, Chandler MJ. Reproductive risk and the continuum of caretaking casualty. In: Horowitz FD, Hetherington EM, Scarr-Salapatek S, Siegel G, eds. *Review of Child Development Research.* Chicago, Ill: University of Chicago Press; 1975.

5. Field TM, Widmayer SM, Stringer S, Ignatoff E. Teenage, lower-class black mothers and their preterm infants. *Child Dev.* 1980;51:426–436.
6. Osofsky JD, Culp AM, Ware LM. Intervention challenges with adolescent mothers and their babies. *Psychiatry.* 1988;51:236–241.
7. Panzarine A. Interpersonal problem solving and its relation to adolescent mothering behaviors. *J Adolesc Res.* 1989;4:53–74.
8. Osofsky JD. Risk and protective factors for teenage mothers and their infants. *Newsl SRCD.* Winter 1990: 1–2.
9. Field TM. Interactions of preterm and term infants with their lower- and middle-class teenage and adult mothers. In: Field TM, Goldberg S, Stern D, Sostek A, eds. *High Risk Infants and Children: Adult and Peer Interactions.* New York, NY: Academic Press; 1980.
10. Reis JA. Comparison of young teenage, older teenage, and adult mothers on determinants of parenting. *J Psychol.* 1988;123:141–151.
11. Stevens JH, Duffield BN. Age and parenting skill among black women in poverty. *Early Child Res Q.* 1986;1:221–235.
12. Gottwald SR, Thurman SK. Parent-infant interaction in neonatal intensive care units: implications for research and service delivery. *Infants Young Child.* 1990;2:1–9.
13. Lawson KR, Daum C, Turkowitz G. Environmental characteristics of neonatal intensive care units. *Child Dev.* 1977;48:1633–1639.
14. Linn PL, Horowitz FD, Buddin BJ, Leake JC, Fox HA. An ecological description of a neonatal intensive care unit. In: Gottfried AW, Gaiter JL, eds. *Infant Stress under Intensive Care.* Baltimore, Md: University Park Press; 1985.
15. Minde KK, Marton P, Manning D, Hines B. Some determinants of mother-infant interaction in the premature nursery. *J Am Acad Child Psychol.* 1980;19:1–21.
16. Rosenfield AG. Visiting the intensive care nursery. *Child Dev.* 1980;51:939–941.
17. Minde KK, Trehub S, Corter C, Boukydis C, Celhoffer L, Marton P. Mother-child relationships in the premature nursery. *Pediatrics.* 1978;61:373–379.
18. Leifer A, Leiderman P, Barnett C, Williams J. Effects of mother-infant separation on maternal attachment behavior. *Child Dev.* 1972;43:1203–1218.
19. Klaus M, Kennell J, Plumb M, Zuehlke S. Human maternal behavior at the first contact with her young. *Pediatrics.* 1970;46:187–192.
20. DiVitto B, Goldberg S. The effects of newborn medical status on early parent-child interaction. In: Field TM, ed. *Infants Born at Risk: Behavior and Development.* New York, NY: SP Medical and Scientific Books; 1979.
21. Brooks-Gunn J, Lewis M. Temperament and affective interaction in handicapped infants. *J Dev Early Child.* 1982;5:31–41.
22. Greene JG, Fox NA, Lewis M. The relationship between neonatal characteristics and three month mother-infant interaction in high risk infants. *Child Dev.* 1983;54:1286–1296.
23. Crawford JW. Mother-infant interaction in premature and full-term infants. *Child Dev.* 1982;53:957–962.
24. Lester BM, Hoffman J, Brazelton TB. The rhythmic structure of mother-infant interaction in term and preterm infants. *Child Dev.* 1985;56:15–27.
25. Crnic K, Ragozin A, Greenberg M, Robinson N, Basham R. Social interaction and developmental competence of preterm and full-term infants during the first year of life. *Child Dev.* 1983;54: 1199–1210.

26. Field T. Effects of early separation, interactive deficits, and experimental manipulations on mother face-to-face interactions. *Child Dev.* 1977;43:763–771.
27. Cunningham CE, Reular E, Blackwell J, Deck J. Behavioral and linguistic development in the interactions of normal and retarded children with their mothers. *Child Dev.* 1981;52:62–70.
28. Jones CL. Criteria for evaluating infant care environments in hospitals. *J Assoc Care Child Hosp.* 1979;1:3.
29. Yoder PJ. Relationship between degree of infant handicap and clarity of infant cues. *Am J Ment Defic.* 1987;91:639–641.
30. Nielson L. *Adolescence: A Contemporary View.* Orlando, Fla: Harcourt Brace Jovanovich; 1991.
31. Prater LP. Early pregnancy and academic achievement of African American youth. *Except Child.* 1992;59:141–149.
32. Elkind D. *Child Development and Education: A Piagetian Perspective.* New York, NY: Oxford University Press; 1976.
33. Elkind D. *The Child's Reality: Three Developmental Themes.* Hillsdale, NJ: Erlbaum; 1978.
34. Elkind D, Bowen R. Imaginary audience behavior in children and adolescents. *Dev Psychol.* 1980;15:38–44.
35. Adams GR, Gulotta TP. *Adolescent Life Experience.* Pacific Grove, Calif: Brooks-Cole; 1989.
36. Thurman SK, Gonsalves SV, Cohen A, Garro A. Parents and Infants Responding: providing services to low income adolescent mothers and their low birth weight babies. Presented at Children on the Edge: Council for Exceptional Children Topical Conference on At-Risk Children and Youth; November 10–12, 1991; New Orleans, La.
37. Lewis M, Goldberg S. Perceptual-cognitive development in infancy: a generalized expectancy model as a function of mother-infant interaction. *Merrill-Palmer Q.* 1969;15:81–100.
38. Bronnfenbrenner U. Toward an experimental ecology of human development. *Am Psychol.* 1977;32: 513–531.
39. Bronnfenbrenner U. *The Ecology of Human Development: Experiments by Nature and Nurture.* Cambridge, Mass: Harvard University Press; 1979.
40. Thurman SK. The congruence of behavioral ecologies: a model for special education programming. *J Spec Educ.* 1977;11:329–333.
41. Thurman SK. Ecological congruence in the study of families with handicapped parents. In: Thurman SK, ed. *Children of Handicapped Parents: Research and Clinical Perspectives.* New York, NY: Academic Press; 1985.
42. Thurman SK, Widerstrom AH. *Infants and Young Children with Special Needs: A Developmental and Ecological Approach* (2nd ed). Baltimore, Md: Brookes; 1990.

Ethical perspectives on family-centered early intervention

Michele M. Sokoly, MS
Doctoral Student
Department of Psychology and Human Development

Paul R. Dokecki, PhD
Professor of Psychology and Special Education
Associate Director for Policy
John F. Kennedy Center
George Peabody College of Vanderbilt University
Nashville, Tennessee

DESPITE THE expressed willingness of professionals to regard families as partners in the care of children with developmental disabilities, partnership thinking has not always prevailed at the level of practice. Throughout much of the recent history of the human services system, a discrepancy has existed between attitudes guiding early intervention and the goal of strengthening families.[1] Several recent assessments[2–7] have found that human services systems are fragmented and sometimes dehumanizing: Diagnoses have often been deficit oriented, professionals have often held negative or indifferent views toward families with children with disabilities, and there has often been a "hands-off" policy on intervening with the family system. Interventions based in this outlook are treatment focused rather than preventive.

This traditional mindset is cautious about forms of intervention that extend beyond treatment of existing problems, arguing, somewhat paradoxically considering the often unfavorable attitudes toward working with families, that "unnecessary intervention harms both family and state."[7(p226)] Such unnecessary intervention is seen as an invasion of privacy and as a threat to the family's ability to function independently.

Much of the recent literature[8–12] argues against a deficit model of intervention and acknowledges the central role of the family in service delivery. In practice, however, early intervention providers have often manifested a professional mentality that is ambivalent about working with families and that may work against their enablement and empowerment.

To achieve the aim of serving children through strengthening families, we must rethink interventions and professional roles. We must shift from traditional modes of intervention toward more ecologic approaches that emphasize a partnership between parents and professionals.

Hobbs and colleagues[1] presented a value framework for guiding family-centered early interventions. They had the ultimate goal of enhancing both community and human development. Their four-part framework argues that interventions should enhance community, strengthen families, enable parents, and enhance and protect the rights of individual family members. This framework suggests that the current early intervention system is on the right track in moving away from more

Inf Young Children 1992; 4(4): 23–32

traditional approaches that have often emphasized individual treatment and viewed the family as both causing its problems and being incapable of dealing with them.[13]

Dunst et al[3] elaborated the theory behind the values framework of Hobbs et al[1] in applying it to the task of guiding family-centered early intervention. They argued that an intervention system for children with disabilities must focus on expressed family needs. Furthermore, it must be concerned not only that the expressed needs are met but with how they are met when determining the adequacy of an intervention. "In order to enable and empower families, we need a breakdown of typical role relationships: paternalistic approaches must be replaced by partnerships."[3(p9)]

The idea of a partnership—entailing service agencies, professionals, and families—is crucial to achieving a balance of shared responsibility for children with disabilities and their families. Such a partnership requires a shift from valuing the individual to valuing the individual within the family within the community.[7] Partnership thinking yields a rationale for intervening with families in pursuit of the value position of Hobbs et al[1] of the caring and competent society. We thereby balance a "preoccupation with rights with a concern for need."[6(p27)] Social ecologic partnership enables families to draw on their strengths and meet their needs in a way that produces growth and not dependence, empowerment and not enfeeblement.

Part H of Public Law (PL) 102-119, the Individuals with Disabilities Education Act—formerly PL 99-457—provides for early intervention for newborns to 3-year-olds. It challenges public agencies, professionals, and families to begin reframing their conceptions of what principles should guide early intervention. A prominent feature of the law is the intent to strengthen and empower the family.[14] Robert Silverstein, chief counsel of the Senate Subcommittee on the Handicapped, stated, "Congress wanted the language of the bill to reflect our utmost respect for the family. The word 'family' must appear ten or fifteen times throughout this legislation. This was intentional. Congress was trying to say: Respect the family."[14(p4)]

The call for the Individualized Family Services Plan (IFSP) clearly shows this emphasis on the family. The IFSP entails statements of the child's level of development, the family's strengths and needs (resources, priorities, and concerns) as they relate to the child's development, and the specific intervention services necessary to meet the unique needs of the child and family.[14] The requirements stress the involvement of the family in designing the intervention. Thus the focus of PL 102-119 (H), at least in theory, requires a shift in the traditional models of intervention toward the ideal of a partnership aimed at strengthening individuals within families within communities.

Because theory and practice do not always connect, implementation often falls short of policy goals. The character and spirit of PL 102-119 manifest a social ecologic perspective that seeks to encourage a multifaceted partnership among society, the professional, and the family. Implementation of the law, however, and particularly the formulation of the IFSP, will prove difficult if the traditional human services mindset persists in service settings. For the IFSP to become a means of strengthening families, we must seriously reexamine the nature of early intervention and become clear about the nature of the parent–professional transaction.

Early intervention professionals and service providers must, in the words of ethicist Gibson Winter, "reconceive the situation . . . [and] question the accepted ways of doing things."[15(p62)] Ethical reflection provides an underutilized means for helping us understand a discrepancy encountered in changing the traditional service system mindset from where it has been in assessing family needs to where it ought to be.

THE TRADITIONAL SYSTEM: AN ILLUSTRATION

We now attempt to account for an important source of the intervention-related discrepancy just mentioned by looking at the ethical aspects of professional roles, character, and structures of power. We present a situation, identified in our research, that exemplifies missed connections in parent–professional transactions. These missed connections are failures to communicate that hinder the family–professional partnership. We chose this story because it is not a clear-cut example of an unethical action. Rather, it represents an instance of everyday practice that takes on new meanings through a process of ethical reflection.

Robb J, 6 months old, was born 2 months prematurely and given only a 5% chance of surviving. He experienced a severe brain hemorrhage at birth, which may have caused a major yet undetermined amount of brian damage. In addition, he had congestive heart failure; swelling around the brain, heart, and lungs; and superventricular tachycardia (his heart beat at twice the normal rate).

His parents are trying to be realistic about Robbie's limitations, are conscientious about finding the best care available for Robbie, and are doing all they can to help him develop to his fullest potential.

They began an early intervention program when Robbie was 4 months old and are seeking the help of many health care and early intervention professionals. They realize that there are no guarantees about the future: No one can say with accuracy what Robbie will be like in 1 year, and the 5-year or 10-year outlook is highly uncertain.

Recently, a neurologist informed the parents that Robbie probably would not develop cerebral palsy. The mother's predictable reaction of elation, however, elicited disparaging comments from the neurologist. "You must remember that cerebral palsy is just a small part of the coin," the mother reported him saying. "We need to concern ourselves with Robbie's mental capacity."

Robbie's mother experienced a profound sense of frustration and of being misunderstood. She tried to appreciate the neurologist's position—he wanted her to realize that much more than cerebral palsy was involved—but she felt that he did not have an accurate sense of what this news really meant to her and her family. One of their major fears, that her son would have to be "strapped in a wheelchair with his head hanging down and his arms and legs straight out," was apparently disconfirmed. Although she understood that this was but one dimension in the complete picture of Robbie's handicaps, she still viewed it as an occasion to celebrate: "When someone gives a parent a white piece of paper, paints it all black, and someone else comes along and throws a little white spot on it, a parent is going to take that spot and milk it for all it's worth." She felt that this was not being unrealistic about the future but rather expressing appreciation and hope in the present moment.

In evaluating her exchange with the neurologist, Robbie's mother concluded "You just have to consider the source. After all, he is a professional."

What went wrong in this encounter between Robbie's mother and his neurologist? Wasn't the neurologist only looking out for the best interest of the family in trying to keep the parents from having unrealistic expectations simply because their multiply handicapped child apparently did not have cerebral palsy? Why then did Mrs J feel so frustrated and misunderstood in this encounter? And what did she mean by her final statement about professionals? Is this the kind of encounter (and our concern here is not only with neurology but with all the early intervention professions) that will lead to empowering relationships or even to the family's receiving needed help?

A MODEL OF PROFESSIONAL ETHICS

Our aim in presenting this situation is to show how current perspectives in ethical theory bear on practice. The appeal to ethics and values is often made only in crisis situations, yet we wish to show in this ordinary example that everyday work with families of children with developmental disabilities is fraught with value issues.

Lebacqz[16] provides an ethical framework that allows fruitful examination of many questions facing the early intervention field. She argues that an adequate approach to ethical discernment, decision, and action requires (1) defining and interpreting the intervention situation in light of duty-based, morally relevant features and professional role expectations; (2) examining the character of the professional; and (3) analyzing the structures of power that influence interventions in actual situations of professional practice. This framework has the potential not only for addressing the specific issues raised by our example but also for suggesting an approach that would both empower and liberate families in pursuit of community and human development, aspects of the vision of the caring and competent society propounded by Hobbs et al.[1]

Situational demands and role expectations

Lebacqz[16] argues that ethical action requires discernment: the capacity to evaluate a situation, to find out its morally relevant features, and to decide why these features are important. Discernment enables us to see what our obligations and decisions are relative to problem setting: choosing to focus on this rather than that aspect of a situation as a problem, framing the reality of that problem, and defining the problem. The traditional case number approach that has often characterized work with families, therefore, is ethically troublesome. The case number approach fails to treat each family as unique and to understand its situation from its perspective, thereby failing to discern the basic values operating in the family system. Professionals must understand these values if they are to be effective helpers.

Perhaps Robbie's mother was frustrated because she felt that her family was treated as a case number. The neurologist was perceived as having a skeptical view of the parents' ability to understand the implications of the child's situation. Although he might have considered it his duty to give the family a realistic picture of Robbie's limitations, he did not discern an equally important duty: to respect the liberty and self-determination of the family. In effect, he gave his opinion, not facts, about the imprecise term *cerebral palsy* and reprimanded the mother for responding to it. As a result, he was perceived as insensitive to the family's value system and as having little faith in their appraisal of their situation. He was viewed as treating the situation as a case needing clarification and not relating to family members as persons. People felt as though they were being treated as things.

The basis for the case number approach is professional role expectations. According to Lebacqz,[16] we think about our obligations in terms of our roles and develop notions of how we should act around others. "Roles provide a link between factual statements about what the situation is and normative assumptions about what the actors ought to do."[16(p36)] The questions, then, are the following: What are the role expectations of professionals and family members involved in the early intervention process? What does each party expect from the other? What should we do?

"An enabling approach to working with families," according to Johnson et al, "requires that professionals reexamine their traditional roles and practices and develop new practices when necessary."[17(p2)] It is this sort of reexamination or reflection on role expectations that Schön[18] has called for. Schön describes two different models of professional roles: model I, technical rationality, and model II, reflection-in-action.

Technical rationality is "the model that is embedded in the institutional context of professional life."[18(p25)] In model I, the professional role centers on problem solving. Problem setting, or the "process by which we define decisions, ends and means, is ignored."[18(p39)] A danger clearly inherent in this model I approach is arbitrarily cutting the practice situation to conform to professional knowledge, which is precisely what occurs when professionals apply a case number approach to family interventions. The professional assumes the role of the expert, the one with all the knowledge. The expectation is that parents will "put themselves in the professionals' hands and comply completely with their advice."[18(p302)] Therefore, model I brings us back to the traditional treatment-focused, top-down approach to interventions: The professional has all the power and all the answers; his or her role is to fix the individual client.

In contrast, reflection-in-action derives from a reframing of the role expectations for both the professionals and the parents. Model II calls for complementarity: The parent and the professional enter a partnership that involves joint exploration of the family's situation. The professional has some expertise, yet he or she realizes that his or her knowledge is incomplete without the unique perspective of the parent. The professional's relationship with the parent "takes on the form of a reflective conversation, where the reflective practitioner tries to discover the limits of his expertise"[18(p300)] instead of imposing predetermined knowledge upon the parent. The model II professional role requires "double vision": The professional as inquirer must "(1) impose an order of his own on the situation, (2) take responsibility for the order he imposes, (3) hold himself open, at the same time he imposes order, to the situation's 'back talk,' "[18(p163)]

Model II's reflective practitioner enters transactions with parents possessing some expert knowledge and a theory of intervention. Unlike the model I professional, however, the reflective practitioner does not assume the traditional expert role. Instead, he or she enters a reflective relationship with the parent that involves exploring multiple perspectives and sharing responsibility for problem setting and problem solving. The early intervention partnership "incorporates recognition of the autonomy of those being served but also includes solidarity with them."[16(p57)]

Professional character

The second dimension of Lebacqz's[16] ethical framework involves character. Professionals must ask themselves not only "What are we to do?" but also "Who are we?"[16(p89)] Their actions over time must somehow be a whole, a story that makes sense and has coherence. The questions for us, therefore, become the following: What should the professional as reflective practitioner be like? What should his or her story be?

According to Lebacqz,[16] codes of professional ethics serve several purposes, an important one being to provide an ideal of professional life. This ideal often suggests that the professional should be "(1) fair, (2) competent, (3) honest, (4) oriented toward the good of the client, and (5) not taking advantage of clients."[16(p70)] This list of characteristics points toward two virtues central to professional life: trustworthiness and prudence.

The professional person as trustworthy trustee deals with issues at the deepest level. This role implies the ability to perceive the family's system of meanings and to understand the intervention situation from the family's perspective. It means sharing responsibility with the parents so that they may maintain, or come to gain, power over their lives.

Related to trustworthiness is prudence, which Lebacqz defines as "the perfected ability to make the right decision." It allows "letting the truth of real things determine what we do."[16(p104)] Prudence entails arriving at good reasons for engaging in interventions through a process of perceiving the situation accurately, deliberating about it wisely, deciding what to do, and acting on that decision. The prudent professional can make the right decision by inviting parents to assume an active role in defining their problems and exploring avenues for intervention.

Central to Lebacqz's[16] portrait of the professional is caring, "a process, a way of relating to someone," argues Mayeroff," that involves [growth and] development."[19(p1)] For professionals to care, they must have not only expertise and knowledge about the other but also self-awareness that allows them to evaluate whether what they are doing helps or hinders the growth of the other. They must "know who the other is, what his power and limitations are, and what is conducive to his growth; [they] must know how to respond to his needs, and what [their] own power and limitations are."[19(p13)] Clearly, the caring professional fulfills the role of reflective practitioner.

To care for the other, the professional must be "*with* the other in his world. He must be able to see from 'inside' what life is like."[19(p42)] Caring professionals treat each situation as unique and allow the "other's growth to guide what [they] do, to help determine how to respond and what is relevant to such a response."[19(p7)] Both these ideas are inherent in the role of the reflective practitioner as trustworthy trustee who prudently approaches families as active partners in a growth-producing process rather than as patients (literally, "passive ones") who need to be cured.

This description of professional character is a departure from the model that has traditionally guided interventions and from the portrait of the neurologist presented in our case. It is stretching the issue to call our neurologist unethical. He apparently intended his remarks to promote the good of the parents by making sure they did not develop unrealistic expectations for their child. The transaction with the family, however, was of questionable validity and effectiveness. Unlike the caring, prudent, and trustworthy professional, the neurologist was perceived as being unaware of the family's perspective, and consequently the transaction resulted in frustration rather than development. Instead of communicating that he was a partner who was on the family's side, he was perceived as callous and insensitive, operating as a model I technically rational expert with all the answers. As this example illustrates, the character of the professional may play a crucial role in parent–professional transactions.

The structure of power

We have described the role of the professional and the character required to perform ethical duties in specific intervention situations. What remains an issue, however, is how to promote such character development and role expectations within the general institutional structure of society and in the structure and design of early intervention programs. The distribution of power is the third part of Lebacqz's[16] ethical framework.

Society vests professionals, by virtue of their role, with authority. Professional power is "legitimated and institutionalized power."[16(p113)] Professionals do not simply have the power to fix a problem. They also define its reality. There is potential for distortion depending upon the way professionals use their reality-defining power.

Craig and Craig argue that differences in the way people exert power stem "from differences in their basic attitudes toward their fellows," whether they "value and cherish" others or see them merely as objects.[20(p59)] They describe two different views of power, labeled directive and synergic. Directive power is "the capacity for an individual to increase his satisfactions by intentionally affecting the behavior of others."[20(p60)] Professionals who operate from this power perspective resemble Schön's[18] model I expert. They use their expert power to exercise control over the other. In doing so, they make the other dependent and powerless: "Directive power dehumanizes people because it makes them less sensitive to the fact that they cause the results of their actions."[20(p61)] Directive power, however, is the sort of power embedded within the structures of society. If we approach families from this unfortunately typical structure of power, we will rarely achieve family enablement and empowerment.

In contrast to directive power, synergic power suggests a different view of professional power. Synergic power is "the capacity of an individual to increase the satisfaction of all participants by intentionally generating increased energy and creativity, all of which is used to *co-create* a more rewarding present and future."[20(p62)] Operating from this model, parents are colleagues and allies with whom professionals join in a cooperative relationship. Synergic power grows from openness and trust. Its ultimate goals are "(1) to increase people's sense of autonomy [as well as] their sense of interdependence [that grows out of working together], (2) to increase their understanding of how they can and do affect their own destiny and the destiny of others, and (3) to build their confidence in people's capacity to work together effectively."[29(p100)] Synergic power counters the traditional views of the professional as controlling expert, and it is this type of power that the caring professional would employ in his or her role as reflective practitioner.

This concept of synergic power also directly relates to issues raised by Lebacqz[16] about the distribution of power. She insists that professionals must seek to share power and redistribute it, yet she recognizes a complex paradox in notions such as empowerment and liberation. If professionals assume that their role is to empower or liberate families, they may come "dangerously close to the trap of paternalism."[16(p131)] The professional's use of power, therefore, must involve synergic efforts, "the working *together* of unlike elements [professionals and parents] to create desirable results unobtainable from any combination of independent efforts."[16(p59)]

The model II professional should not ask "What can I *do* for this parent?" but rather "How would liberation happen here?" Synergic rather than directive transactions with families have a much greater chance of addressing families' real needs and priorities, equalizing the distribution of power, and promoting community and human development.

In our example, the professional structures operating in the transaction with the J family were perceived as entailing the exercise of directive power. The traditional role of the physician is to cure, to give patients directions about what to do to improve their conditions. With a child with disabilities, however, there is no cure, no one prescription that will heal all ailments. The neurologist was viewed as not making this distinction and as operating directively: He offered his evaluation of the child's condition—"It is highly unlikely that Robbie will develop cerebral palsy"—predicting the child's uncertain future development. When Robbie's mother reacted positively to this news, the neurologist was seen as seeking to direct her to a realistic assessment of the situation, emphasizing deficits and ignoring strengths rather than understanding the family's underlying value system. The parent and professional did not jointly explore the problem; instead, the professional was seen as controlling the balance of power and knowledge by virtue of his professional status.

For synergic power to operate, an alternative type of relationship must replace the paternalistic relationship operating in our example. We refer here to the we-relation, a concept described by Alfred Schutz and expanded by Winter.[15] The we-relation entails interdependence of self and other as persons, not things, It involves "being conscious of the other by grasping the other's meaning."[15(p104)] According to Winter, the "decisive criterion for the meaning of action is the project of the actor."[15(p131)] The work of the professional, therefore, is to explore and understand, in partnership with family members, the nature of family projects; the task is not to impose meaning upon families by the exercise of directive or coercive power. In effect, our analysis suggests that a basic aspect of ethics entails human beings transacting as persons, not as things.[21–25]

APPLYING ETHICAL THEORY TO PRACTICE

Now that we have developed an ethical theory of parent–professional transactions on the basis of conceptualizations of the professional's role, character, and exercise of power, we must explore ways of translating this theory into practice. How can professionals assume the role of reflective practitioners, develop a character of caring, and exercise synergic power?

If the parent–professional transaction entails the we-relation, one of the key elements becomes identifying and defining family projects as opposed to assessing family needs and strengths. According to the model of reflective practice, the task of formulating an IFSP should promote understanding between parents and professionals, creating a synthesis of family resources, priorities, concerns, and projects on the one hand and professional expertise on the other. The key to developing such an understanding lies in parent–professional communication.[26,27] Critical theory, as proposed by Habermas and expanded by Forrester,[28,29] provides a means for analyzing communication in pursuit of the ideal of "uncoerced consensus and nonmanipulated understanding and agreement."[29(p238)] This ideal relates to the concept of synergic power by emphasizing working together to formulate intervention plans instead of imposing interventions upon families. It also provides a means of coming to know the family situation, which is a central part of the caring transaction.

Critical theory identifies obstacles that impede communication and prevent parents and professionals from jointly exploring family projects and meanings. According to Forrester's model of communication, claims to the validity of what "speakers and listeners . . . say and hear" must be considered.[29(p236)] Listeners evaluate four claims in what they hear: (1) truth, the existence of some state of affairs; (2) legitimacy, the appropriateness of what they hear in the context in which they hear it; (3) sincerity, whether they believe the speaker means and intends to say what he or she is saying; and (4) clarity, the comprehensibility and coherence of what is being said.

Acceptance of these communicative claims has pragmatic results. The claim to truth engenders belief, legitimacy engenders consent, sincerity engenders trust, and clarity engenders attention. On the other hand, when these claims are distorted, misinformation and manipulation may result. Several examples of these communicative claims and their violation can be drawn from situations involving parent–professional transactions in early intervention.

When early intervention agents do not provide parents with honest information about the condition of their child and deny developmental concerns that do exist, the claim to truth is invalidated. When parents see delays in development that call into question their beliefs about their child's normality, they may begin to doubt any information they receive from the intervention agent. This would have serious effects on the parent–professional relationship because channels of communication and discourse have broken down. Similar problems result when any of the other communicative claims are denied.

The claim of legitimacy involves issues such as whether professionals have adequate information about child and family resources, priorities, concerns, and projects to plan useful early interventions. Although parents might verbally consent to illegitimate recommendations, they are not likely to be able to carry them out.

If the claim of sincerity is not upheld, cooperation and trust cannot be maintained. Attempts by professionals to manipulate information and misguide parents' judgments about their children would invalidate this claim.

Finally, the claim to clarity relates to whether professionals communicate with parents in readily understandable, jargon-free language. If this is not so, parents might leave the professional's office feeling confused and frustrated.

In contrast to these examples, honoring claims to communication has the potential to lead to authentic partnership and to produce more effective interventions. Because of the importance of upholding the validity of communicative claims, free and uncoerced communication becomes a necessity in parent–professional transactions. "As discourse is denied to participants, they are likely to be rendered dependent, powerless, ignorant, and mystified."[29(p240)] This suggests that the answer to Lebacqz's[16] question "How would liberation happen here?" involves eliminating socially unnecessary distortions in communication between parents and professionals. Forrester[28,29] asserts that some distortions, those that are accidental and unforeseeable, are bound to occur; however, others are neither natural nor socially necessary, and as a result are avoidable. These socially unnecessary distortions probably occur when professionals assume an imperious expert role, are insensitive and impersonal, and use directive power to exert control over families. Communication and power dynamics, of course, will play out differently in specific situations.

Problems in communication were at the heart of what went wrong in the specific transaction involving Robbie and his family. The communication context was distorted because the professional was perceived as not taking the time to establish the kind of relationship with family members that allowed him to understand their interpretation of the situation. Although he attempted to uphold the claim to truth by not withholding information from Robbie's parents, his remarks were incomplete and distorting and were viewed as neither legitimate nor appropriate in the context of how the family was coming to terms with Robbie's handicaps. The parents had already accepted Robbie's limitations and wanted to have the chance to be happy at the ray of hope given when they found out he probably would not develop cerebral palsy and might someday be able to walk. The neurologist, perceived as assuming a traditional, paternalistic approach, made the family feel that they could not count on him as a partner. This approach is problematic for promoting the ends of community and human development.

• • •

Our ethical analysis suggests that professionals involved in early intervention and formulating IFSPs must assume the role of the reflective practitioner, embody a caring and prudent character as trustworthy trustee, and operate on the basis of synergic power that flows out of the we-relation. Furthermore, they must engage in a process of free and uncoerced communication with families, which allows family projects and underlying family values to be identified.

This view of parent–professional transactions requires a shift from the traditional case number, paternalistic, and model I expert model, in which family members are treated as things, not persons. It is only through such a shift in conceptualizing parent–professional transactions that the goal of liberating, empowering, and enabling families with children with disabilities will be accomplished. The recent movement of the early intervention field in this direction has the potential to keep IFSPs from becoming simply mandated paperwork and opportunities for experts to exert directive and coercive power over families.

Concluding with a few specifics, we draw the following implications from our ethical analysis for IFSP practice:

1. Partnership that encourages active involvement of all participants must characterize the fashioning of IFSPs. This focus on working in partnership will require both family members and early intervention professionals to redefine roles and change expectations.
2. The atmosphere of the IFSP meeting should encourage open dialogue and sharing of information, what we have been calling free and uncoerced communication. In that regard, professionals should be open to parents' questions and comments and should beware of too readily interpreting them as hostile, defensive, or as evidence of resistance.
3. The structure of the IFSP meeting should be flexible enough to enable each family to express its unique value system, story, and project.

REFERENCES

1. Hobbs N, Dokecki PR, Hoover-Dempsey KV, Moroney RM, Shayne MW, Weeks KH. *Strengthening Families.* San Francisco, Calif: Jossey-Bass; 1984.
2. Dokecki PR. A family perspective of evaluating children's behavioral health services. Paper presented at the conference on Children's Behavioral Health Initiative; June 1989; Tempe, Ariz.
3. Dunst CJ, Trivette CM, Deal AG. *Enabling and Empowering Families.* Cambridge, Mass: Brookline; 1988.
4. Heflinger CA. *Bridging the Gap between Policy Enactment and Street Level Implementation of PL 99-457 and Related Early Intervention Programs for Young Children with Handicapping Conditions and Their Families.* Nashville, Tenn: Vanderbilt University; 1989. Thesis.
5. Kaiser AP, Hemmeter ML. Value based approaches to family intervention. *Top Early Child Spec Ed.* 1989;8:72–86.
6. Moroney RM. Shared responsibility: For whose benefit and for what purpose? In: Nottingham J, Nottingham J, eds. *The Professional and Family Caregiver: Dilemmas, Rewards, and New Directions.* Americus, Ga: Georgia Southwestern College; 1990.

7. Moroney RM, Dokecki PR. The family and the professions: Implications for public policy. *J Fam Issues.* 1984;5:224–238.
8. Bailey DB. Issues and perspectives in family assessment. *Infants Young Child.* 1991;4:26–34.
9. Weissbourd B, Kagan SL. Family support programs: Catalysts for change. *Am J Orthopsychiatr.* 1989;59:20–31.
10. Zigler E, Berman W. Discerning the future of early childhood intervention. *Am Psychol.* 1983;38:894–906.
11. Zigler E, Black KB. America's family support movement: Strengths and limitations. *Am J Orthopsychiatr.* 1989;59:6–19.
12. Zigler E, Seitz V. Early childhood intervention programs: A reanalysis. *Sch Psychol Rev.* 1980;9:354–368.
13. Moroney RM. *Shared Responsibility: Families and Social Policy.* New York, NY: Aldine; 1986.
14. Gallagher J, Place P, Shields M. *The Generation of Policy Options: The Family.* Chapel Hill, NC: Carolina Policy Studies Program; 1989.
15. Winter G. *Elements for a Social Ethic: The Role of Social Science in Social Policy.* New York, NY: Macmillan; 1966.
16. Lebacqz K. *Professional Ethics: Power and Paradox.* Nashville, Tenn: Abingdon; 1985.
17. Johnson BH, McGonigel MJ, Kaufman RK. *Guidelines and Recommended Practices for the Individualized Family Services Plan.* Washington, DC: Association for the Care of Children's Health; 1989.
18. Schön DA. *The Reflective Practitioner: How Professionals Think in Action.* New York, NY: Basic Books; 1983.
19. Mayeroff M. *On Caring.* New York, NY: Harper & Row; 1971.
20. Craig JH, Craig M. *Synergic Power: Beyond Domination and Submissiveness.* Berkeley, Calif: Proactive Press; 1973.
21. Dokecki PR. On knowing the person as agent in caring relation. *Person-Centered Rev.* 1990;5:155–169.
22. Dokecki PR. On knowing the community of caring persons: A methodological basis for the reflective-generative practice of community psychology. *J Community Psychol.* 1992;20:26–35.
23. Kirkpatrick FG. *Community: A Trinity of Models.* Washington, DC: Georgetown University Press; 1986.
24. Macmurray J. *The Self as Agent.* London, England: Faber; 1957.
25. Macmurray J. *Persons in Relation.* New York, NY: Harper & Bros; 1961.
26. Able H. *Parent-Professional Communication Relative to Medical Care Decision Making for Seriously Ill Newborns.* Nashville, Tenn: Vanderbilt University; 1986. Thesis.
27. Able-Boone H, Dokecki PR, Smith MS. Parent and health care provider communication and decision making in the intensive care nursery. *Child Health Care.* 1989;18:133–141.
28. Forrester J. Planning the face of power. *J Am Plann Assoc.* 1982;48:67–80.
29. Forrester J. Critical theory and organizational analysis. In: Morgan G, ed. *Beyond Method: Strategies for Social Research.* Beverly Hills, Calif: Sage; 1983.

In the best interest of the family: The emergence of family resource programs

Bernice Weissbourd, MA
President

Maureen Patrick, MA
Executive Director
Family Focus
Evanston, Illinois

THE TERMS "family support" and "family resource" are becoming increasingly familiar as programs bearing those or similar names begin to dot the American landscape. State and federal legislation for children's programs now include family support components. Public schools, in their move toward serving very young children, are including family support programs. Developmental disabilities organizations are promoting family support services, such as respite care, cash subsidy, special recreation opportunities, and self-advocacy training.

The term family support is often confusing, having different meanings for different social-service disciplines. In the wide spectrum of social services, family support refers to programs that enable families to stay together after a crisis. The emerging view is that support for families should be available on a continuum from prevention through early intervention to crisis management and long-term supportive measures. In the context of this article, family support refers to the first of the programs on this continuum: preventive programs designed to help families before they are in crisis; to reach all families; and to reflect the strengths, needs, and culture of the families for whom they exist. Although the terms are used interchangeably, the authors call such support "family resource programs."

This article describes the history, the principles that drive program implementation, and the essential features of family resource programs that distinguish them from other services. Also presented are ways in which families with children who are developmentally disabled (or at risk for disability) can benefit from involvement in mainstream family resource programs and suggest implications for practitioners of expanding the concept of community integration of persons with developmental disabilities into family resource programs.

HISTORICAL PERSPECTIVE

A brief history of the origins of family resource programs will shed light on some of the characteristics they share.[1] One of the roots of these programs is in the informational focus of parent education. In this country, parent education evolved from the informal process of sharing child-rearing information to organized associations of parents seeking an understanding of the best ways to rear their children. Family resource programs reflect the goal in parent education of informing parents about the most current knowledge of principles in child development.

Inf Young Children 1988; 1(2): 46–54

The roots of family resource programs can also be traced to the self-help movement that flourished in the 1960s. Belonging to a group of people sharing a similar interest or problem became an acceptable way of acknowledging interdependence, an important antecedent for family resource programs. Even in the early 1950s, the emergence of grass-roots organizations of parents of mentally retarded children in communities throughout the United States led to the formation of the Associations for Retarded Citizens. ARC became a model for community-based advocacy and support organizations, and it demonstrated the political power of coalitions of parents working for services for their children.

While parent education, self-help, and political empowerment are prominent themes in the history of family resource development, another major contribution comes from a very different model of social service: the settlement house. Strengthening neighborhood and family life, the clarion call of settlement houses, is echoed in the stated goals of family resource programs. The settlement house view that the family and its fortunes are interrelated with the life of the community and the social policies of the nation is intimately connected with the ecologic approach of many family resource programs.

Most recently, Head Start and Parent–Child Development Centers have demonstrated the significance of parent involvement in fostering the development of their children.[2] Through Head Start, parents who had limited access to child development information and who had not felt any measure of control over the institutions that served their children were able to exert some power over the content and direction of early childhood programs. The need for information and the desire to feel empowered remain a significant motivation for participation in family resource programs.

In the mid 1970s, family resource programs emerged from these varied roots and as a result of the particular climate of the period. The social values, economic realities, and personal needs that families faced in that time of rapid change were qualitatively different from those that confronted previous generations. These changes, which continue today, include the increasing percentage of mothers in the work force; the changes in family structure brought about by divorce, remarriage, and single parenthood; the increasing geographic mobility of families; and the growing poverty among children, particularly those in female-headed households. The climate was right for the emergence of an entirely new kind of program based, in part, on older forms, but reflecting the desire to support family life through a community of people with similar concerns.

Though family resource programs may have common roots, the diversity of programs defies simple explanations. The programs come in every shape and size; they exist in almost every kind of community and under every kind of auspice. They are located in community centers, schools, churches, the workplace, homes, store-fronts, or wherever it is convenient for families to meet. In many cases, traditional social service agencies—child care centers, mental health centers, Head Start programs, or health clinics, for example—have added family resource components to their existing programs. In other instances, families themselves have organized cooperative support groups and meet in each other's homes. School systems are incorporating family resource programs, and human services departments in some states are including prevention-oriented family support programs as integral parts of their systems.

The array of services provided by family resource programs is as varied as their strengths,[3] which are described in *Programs to Strengthen Families: A Resource Guide,* available from the Family Resource Coalition, 230 North Michigan Avenue, Suite 1625, Chicago, IL 60601. The services are largely determined by the needs and desires of the parents in the community; by the fiscal, professional, and volunteer resources available; and by the program goals of the sponsoring agency. At one end of the spectrum of services are comprehensive, community-based programs ranging from drop-in times to crisis intervention, parent education, support groups, home visitors, information and referral, and parent advocacy. These programs tend to function as community centers for families. At the other end are single-focused programs, such as "warm lines" that provide telephone information on child development, or a parent education course based on a specific curriculum given in a time-limited period. In between are self-help, mutual-aid types of parent support groups, some focused on parents of children with special needs.

GUIDING PRINCIPLES

The dominant principles underlying the growing family resource movement distinguish these programs from other social services. In contrast to social service delivery systems oriented toward ameliorating crisis, family resource programs reflect the following basic assumptions:

- focus on prevention,
- recognition of the importance of the early years,
- ecologic approach,
- holistic view of the parent as a total person, and
- value of support.

Focus on prevention

Programs are primarily oriented toward prevention of families' and children's problems rather than focusing on treatment. The prevention approach extends beyond simply avoiding a predictable problem to a concept of "optimalism."

Optimalism means providing an environment conducive to the optimal development of children through support of the family and maintenance of a viable community. For children with developmental disabilities, family resource programs may seek to reduce the risk of institutionalization; to promote integration of the child and family with the larger community, thus reducing their isolation; and to enable the family as a group and as individuals to engage in a wide range of interests and pursuits.

A focus on prevention in this context has broad implications for how services are perceived and delivered. If prevention is providing an optimal environment in which children can grow and develop into as healthy adults as possible, it does, by necessity, mean serving all families. Since it is impossible to know who may experience problems as they grow, everyone becomes the target population. This approach assumes universal access, regardless of economic status, race, ethnicity, ability, or disability. A belief in prevention makes claims on the society to ensure a baseline of good beginnings for all children because it is their right, not because problems are prevented or that services may prove to be cost-effective.

Recognition of the importance of the early years

The implications of positive experiences and good attachments in the very early years for cognitive, emotional, and social development are evident in the extensive research on infants and toddlers. Closely allied to a preventive approach is the availability of programs to support parents from pregnancy through their child's early years, to prepare parents before the birth of their child, and to assist the establishment of an optimal reciprocal relationship between parents and infants. Though getting the right start is no insurance against future problems, it does lay the groundwork for good development, which alleviates the necessity for early remedial measures.

Ecologic approach

Because "the family is the most effective and economical system for fostering and sustaining the development of the children,"[4(p595)] children cannot be seen as separate from the family and community in which they live. Family resource programs mark a move from a child-centered to a family–community-centered approach. The validity of this shift in emphasis is evidenced in research[4] indicating that programs working with children and parents are more effective than programs working with children alone.

Since an ecologic approach assumes that the community is integral to the life of the family, a sensitivity to the cultural and social traditions of a community is an essential element in family resource programs. Programs are based on the awareness that parents are products of their cultures, and their child-rearing patterns reflect their culture's customs and traditions.

Programs not only reflect the community, they also build the community. "Some of these programs may strengthen the bonds among people in the community, thereby increasing the availability of informal support and enriching the community environment for families."[5(p148)]

Holistic view of the parent as a total person

"The child is father to the man" is a familiar adage now reinforced by knowledge that parental behavior is influenced by the experience of the parent as a child. Parenthood is described as reexperiencing the past and as a time of reactivating old conflicts and bringing new hopes.[6] Parenthood, viewed in these terms, emphasizes the possibilities for individual growth and development. Such an approach recognizes that parents learn from experience as well as from facts, are more than vessels in which to pour information, and tend to acquire and retain knowledge as it is relevant to their lives.

Parental behavior has a primary influence on the development of children. Parents who are stimulating and express confidence in their child-rearing enhance the child's social and cognitive growth.[7] Research supports the assumption in family support programs that positive feelings of self-worth enable parents to be more effective in their parenting roles. The assumption reinforces the family resource program's focus on the parent as a *total* person.

Value of support

The positive effect of support for families has been well documented, though common sense itself reinforces that conclusion. There is clear evidence that the often devastating results of isolation and loneliness can be alleviated through the development of social networks and that such support is associated with more responsive interaction with children and strengthened coping capacities.[8–10]

In recognizing the necessity of support, the term no longer implies deficits, but, on the contrary, speaks to the strength and capacity of a family to develop friendships, to make linkages with other groups, and to seek advice and information. The fact is support programs increase a family's ability to cope, rather than provide a system on which families become dependent. The empowerment of parents to control their lives and to become involved in shaping their environment at neighborhood and national levels may be a natural result of the experiences parents have in support programs.

PROGRAM CHARACTERISTICS

Emanating from the principles fundamental to family support programs is a unique *set* of characteristics. Family resource programs represent a new form of service, new staff roles and relationships, and new patterns of decision making.

Range of services

Unlike traditional services focusing on specific problem areas, family resource programs recognize the necessity for a range of services. Program planners are challenged to find the particular kind of support from which a family can benefit.[11] Services most frequently provided by family resource programs are parenting and child development education, support groups for parents, drop-in centers, information and referral services, peer support, parent–child joint activities, health and nutrition education, and warm lines.

Staffing pattern and professional role

One of the major contributions to the family support field is the innovative staffing pattern and professional roles that have been explored and used in family resource programs. The traditional role of the professional as the expert and final authority no longer fits in a program where parents are seen as total people, as advocates on their own behalf, and as the most significant influence in the child's life. The roles of teacher–learner or therapist–patient or authority–client change to one in which knowledge is shared between parents and professionals, and parents and professionals together determine program design and direction. The strengths of parents are recognized and built on, and the expertise of professionals is utilized in an atmosphere of mutuality, respect, and shared problem solving. Whittaker and Garbarino suggest that the key implication of this increasing trend toward partnership with parents is that the field will quite literally never be the same again.[12]

When the focus is not on diagnosis and treatment of the individual, but on an understanding of the child and family in relation to their environment, staff must know the community in ways not typical of other services. It is not sufficient for staff to know community resources and how parents can connect with them. They must also know the cultural traditions, the expectations, and the child-rearing patterns of the community. Consequently, staff sensitivity to the community often sets the tone for the staff–parent relationship.

Health model

Using a nondeficit model to approach the goal of nurturing families to function more effectively challenges program designers to build on strengths—not merely manage the deficits—of the families they serve. Programs are planned to start with the strengths that families already have. Parents' sense of self is enhanced as the skills of parents are used in program planning and operations and as opportunities for leadership are structured into program designs. Staff members assume strength of some kind in every family; therefore, the silent question asked about families is no longer "What's their problem?" but "What do they have going for them?"

Responsiveness to community

Family resource programs are found in communities of every income level and ethnic and racial composition. The characteristics of the family in the community determine specific program direction and structure. Parents in middle-class communities seek out programs to alleviate the isolation and loneliness prevalent in a society where families are separated by geographic distances, and resources for child-rearing advice and support are seldom present. Friendships and peer groups provide emotional and concrete support (baby-sitting co-ops, clothing exchanges, etc), while information on child development relieves the intense anxiety over "Is what I am doing right?"

In immigrant communities, parents rely on family resource programs to help them become familiar with the customs of a strange culture, with a new language, with the institutions with which they must deal. They learn the child-rearing patterns and expectations of a society different from theirs; and with that knowledge, they can determine how much of the new to accept and which of the older traditions to retain.

Low-income communities, often including families whom poverty has put at high-risk, require, in addition to informal social support important to the families' well-being, a more focused intervention that would address specific obstacles to adequate parenting.[13]

INTEGRATION OF FAMILIES WITH SPECIAL NEEDS

The resources of a family support program can be deeply meaningful to a family that daily faces an uncertain future for itself and for one or more of its children. The assumption that competent caring for children thrives in an environment where parents have healthy self-esteem and a belief in their ability to manage pertains to all families.

In a family resource program, parents and staff together face life's ambiguities. Together they build on the inherent strength of individuals and families, cherish differences, care for and support one another. The sense of community commitment that pervades the family resource movement can be of particular benefit to families with special needs. Since children who have, or are at risk for, one or more disabling conditions will require some specialized services, these should be perceived as an addition, not a substitute for the community-based family resource program.

No family can or should expect to have all of its needs met by the family resource program. Families that frequent a neighborhood resource program may go to different churches, have children in different schools, work in different towns, and come from different parts of the country, but they also share common bonds. These bonds include a desire to foster family development and a belief in each family member's right to develop to his or her fullest potential.

Families with children who have real or potential developmental disabilities are, like any other family, in need of community acceptance and derive enormous benefit from identifying with an organization committed to supporting parental competence. Participation in a family resource program promotes the family's involvement in the general community and prevents the isolation often experienced by families with children who have special needs. Community integration, or mainstreaming, of children with special needs must begin early if the goal of providing developmentally appropriate experiences for all children and families is to be achieved.

The ways that family resource programs support families are as varied as the families who use them. A program can be an integral part of an overall family support plan for children who have special needs. For example, a family with a child who has phenylketonuria (PKU) has several needs. Parents, siblings, and, on occasion, aunts, uncles, and cousins may undergo genetic counseling. The child with PKU requires a precise diet and overall medical management by a highly specialized professional team. PKU support groups offering education about this disorder can help a family learn to deal with complicated health-insurance issues, ways to provide nutritious meals that conform to strict dietary restrictions, and feelings related to carrying a genetic disorder. Genetic counseling, diet, medical management, and educational groups all support the outcome of preventing medical retardation in a child who has PKU. Although the family and child with PKU need these specialized services, they also need to participate in the wider life of their community.

If the child and family are involved early with family resource programs, they can build and practice skills necessary for managing special needs within the context of ordinary community life. The child with PKU, juvenile diabetes, or other conditions requiring special regimens can learn to be comfortable with his or her special needs within the context of everyday interaction in heterogenous groups of children and parents. Thus, in addition to supporting parental competence and decreasing family isolation, family resource programs (1) promote community acceptance of children with, or at risk for, developmental disabilities; (2) enable families whose children have special needs to identify with other families who have different needs; and (3) increase general awareness about handicapping conditions. A current public service advertisement says, "How do you treat a handicapped person? Like a person." How should we treat a family with a child who has a disabling condition? Like a family.

IMPLICATIONS FOR PRACTICE

To learn more about becoming involved with family resource programs:

- Find out about family resource programs serving the communities where your families live. (For information, write to the Family Resource Coalition, 230 N. Michigan Avenue, Suite 1625, Chicago, IL 60601.)
- Visit family resource programs, become familiar with their programs, prepare them for your plans to refer families, and begin a relationship wherein you can be a resource for families of children with special needs.
- Identify other mainstream organizations, such as churches, YMCAs, and park districts, that may work with you to promote integrated family support services. Encourage these entities to remember families with children who have disabilities when they develop family-oriented programs.
- Include referral to family resource programs as part of the individualized support plan for each family with whom you work.
- Join (or form) coalitions of individuals and organizations that promote family resource programs.
- Be knowledgeable about local, state, and federal legislation supporting family resource programs.
- Advocate for expansion and funding for family support programs that reflect the myriad needs, strengths, and structure of American families.
- Find out if there is a Parent Training and Information Center near you. Get on their mailing list and establish a relationship with them.
- Apply the principles of the family resource movement, especially the parent–professional partnership, in all aspects of your work.

• • •

Family resource programs emerged as a response to the changing scene for American families and mark this generation's way of ensuring the family's continuing strength. The rapid growth and expansion of family resource programs in a brief period of approximately 10 to 15 years dramatically attests to the fact that families desire and seek support as a means of alleviating the stress of changing social circumstances or disabling conditions. By fostering parents' sense of worth and competence in an environment in which concerns are shared, parents are able to become advocates on their own behalf, shaping their communities and speaking out on policies affecting their families' ability to function.

Beyond the value of providing early support to prevent problems later, the health model of social services represented by family resource programs underscores a commitment to ensure that all children and families have the opportunity to develop to their fullest potential. In providing the support necessary to assist families to function well from the outset, our nation can change its social service system from one organized primarily to deal with crisis to one organized to prevent it.

As professionals are challenged to think and plan in new directions, a steadily expanding public awareness is encouraging the development of programs to support families in their child-rearing roles. This is truly a time when massive concern for the present crisis for children and families in our country is impelling people from all segments of society—policy makers, corporate leaders, professionals, and parents—to find and implement new solutions.

People who care for and about children and parents can be a strong and effective force for establishing family resource programs throughout the United States. As noted, family resource programs dot the landscape, and landmark programs have begun to emerge and serve as beacons for future development. The response of local, state, and federal governments and corporate communities to secure the existence of family resource programs has yet to be firmly placed on the national agenda. Initial steps have been taken by some states to establish programs, and federal legislation for child care recognizes the importance of including programs for families of the children served. The next steps require guaranteed funding for present and expanded program development, for training personnel, and for continued research on program effectiveness. Family resource programs cannot solve all of the nation's social ills, but they can make a difference in the state of the family and in revitalizing human services.

REFERENCES

1. Kagan SL, Powell DR, Weissbourd B, et al: *America's Family Support Programs.* New Haven, Conn, Yale University Press, 1987.
2. Abt C: The evaluation of social programs. Beverly Hills, Calif, Sage, 1976.
3. *Programs to Strengthen Families: A Resource Guide.* New Haven, Conn, Yale University Bush Center in Child Development and Social Policy, 1983.
4. Bronfenbrenner U: *Is Early Intervention Effective? A Report on Longitudinal Evaluations of Preschool Programs.* US Dept of Health, Education and Welfare Government Printing Office, 1974.
5. Weiss H: Family and education in early childhood programs, in Kagen SL, Powell DR, Weissbourd B, et al (eds): *America's Family Support Programs.* New Haven, Conn, Yale University Press, 1987.

6. Anthony JE, Benedek T (eds): *Parenthood: Its Psychology and Psychopathology.* Boston, Little, Brown, 1970.
7. Clarke-Stewart KA, Apfel N: Evaluating parental effects on child development, in Schulman L. (ed): *Review of Research Education.* Itasca, Ill, Peacock, 1978, vol 6, pp 47–119.
8. Colletta ND: Social support and the risk of maternal rejection by adolescent mothers. *J Psychol* 1981;109:191–197.
9. Crinic KA, Greenburg MT, Ragozin AS, et al: Effects of stress and social support on mothers and premature and full-term infants. *Child Dev* 1983;54:209–217.
10. Wandersman PL, Wandersman A, Kahn S: Social support in the transition to parenthood. *J Commun Psychol* 1980;8(4):332-342.
11. Powell DR: *A Social Interactional Approach to Parent Education: An Overview of the Child and Family Neighborhood Program.* Detroit, Mich, The Merrill-Palmer Institute, 1976.
12. Whittaker JK, Garbarino J, et al: *Social Support Networks: Informal Helping in the Human Services.* New York, Aldine, 1983.
13. Halpern R: Community based support for high-risk young families. *Soc Policy,* Summer 1986.

The individualized family service plan and the early intervention team: Team and family issues and recommended practices

Mary J. McGonigel, MS
Family-Centered Care Project Coordinator
Association for the Care of Children's Health
Washington, DC

Corinne W. Garland, MA
Executive Director
Child Development Resources, Inc.
Lightfoot, Virginia

WHEN PUBLIC LAW 99-457, the Education of the Handicapped Amendments of 1986, was being developed, there was near unanimity within the field of early intervention regarding several critical issues addressed in the nascent bill. This consensus, evident in a Congressional report[1] and in the testimony provided to Congress by leading early intervention organizations and practitioners, extended to the belief that a team approach was necessary and that families were essential members of the team.

The testimony reflected the commonly held belief that the infant is uniquely dependent on the family. This physical and emotional dependence requires that early intervention services be provided within the context of the family. Legislators were urged to specify the role of families in early intervention as both planners and recipients of services and to require written program plans addressing not only the needs of the infant, but also the strengths and needs of the family.

Now that Public Law 99-457 is a reality, no provision is producing more controversy and anxiety than the individualized family service plan (IFSP). Many families and service providers alike are concerned about the potential for an assessment and planning process that will be intrusive, judgmental, static, or unresponsive to the family's needs. Others, more optimistic, are searching for best practices for defining, encouraging, and supporting the family's role on the early intervention team.

This article will define the concepts of team and team interaction as they relate to early intervention, discuss the evolution of the family's role on the team, and suggest principles and practices for team development of the IFSP that are consistent with this new role. Examples of exemplary family-focused principles and practices will be provided.

THE TEAM IN EARLY INTERVENTION

Prior to the passage of Public Law 99-457, a team approach to organizing services for young children with special needs and their families was becoming wide-

Inf Young Children 1988; 1(1): 10–21

spread and was gaining support among early intervention professionals.[2,3] The support was in part a result of Public Law 94-142 and in part a result of the growing recognition that no one discipline can meet the diverse and complex needs of these young children and their families.[4]

No longer an option, a team process now must be used to provide three services required by the new law: team assessment, IFSP development, and case management. Those programs that had resisted the team approach are now examining established models for team organization. Others, already using a team approach, are reexamining the organization of their teams and the ways in which those teams work together.

There are many definitions of a "team." Fewell provides one of the simplest: A team is at least two persons associated through work or activity.[2] This definition encompasses all forms and types of early intervention teams. Common to most definitions of "team organization," however, is the concept of interdependence. Holm and McCartin describe a team as "an interacting group performing integrated and interdependent activities."[5(p121)] Dyer describes teams as "collections of people who must rely on group collaboration if each member is to experience the optimum of success and goal achievement."[6(p4)] To be effective in serving young children with special needs and their families, early intervention teams must be more than collections of persons pursuing their own interests and tasks. The group, "functioning together, is greater than the sum of its individual parts."[7(p306)]

This notion of the team being an interdependent and collaborative group can be actualized only when there is a structure for interaction among team members. Three models for team interaction have been identified and discussed in the early intervention literature: the multidisciplinary, interdisciplinary, and transdisciplinary models.[2,3,8,9]

Much attention has been paid to distinguishing one model from another. A certain controversy has attended the discussion, particularly with regard to the transdisciplinary model, the newest among the models for early intervention teams. While many find the transdisciplinary approach difficult to accept and implement because of the high level of interaction and working across disciplinary boundaries that it requires, proponents consider the results well worth the effort.

It is unfortunate that so much attention has been given to naming and defending models of team interaction. Faced with the challenge of developing IFSPs that are, in fact, neither judgmental nor intrusive, the team's energy would be better spent on increasing the interaction among team members and improving the quality of that interaction.

Only recently have early intervention teams begun to examine their team's functioning systematically. As Fewell cautions, "teams are made, not born."[2(p304)] Early intervention personnel struggling to develop effective teams are experiencing a number of problems that are described in the literature: "differing levels of participation by different occupational groups . . .; lack of meaningful discussion in team meetings . . .; problems in implementing team recommendations . . .; lack of training and guidance in the team process . . .; and the inability of professionals to work together in a truly integrative fashion."[10(p17)]

Bennett[7] and Healy et al[11] add to the list of team problems the higher status traditionally accorded to team members from certain disciplines, particularly medicine. This difference in status and the related difference in personnel costs may be one reason that many early intervention teams outside hospital settings do not include physicians and psychologists. Many concepts such as team building, group process, and team maintenance can be profitably borrowed from the literature of social work, psychology, and organizational development to help early intervention programs overcome these and other team problems.

Teams examining their own structure and function in light of the provisions of Public Law 99-457 and current best practices will be best served by arriving at a consensus about their team's goals and constraints, and then choosing the model of team interaction that allows these goals to be met.

MODELS FOR TEAM INTERACTION

A review of the three most common models for team interaction and their usual procedures for assessment and program planning will be helpful to teams choosing or reevaluating a model for their work. All three models are based on a team made up of professionals from a variety of disciplines, often including education, social work, medicine, physical therapy, occupational therapy, and speech-language pathology. Families of infants and children with special needs are included on these teams in various ways and degrees.

Early intervention teams share a common task: the assessment of a child's developmental status and the development and implementation of a program of services to meet the child's needs. Public Law 99-457 requires that the individualized program plan also be based on the family's assessed needs.

Although the composition and tasks may be quite similar for multidisciplinary, interdisciplinary, and transdisciplinary teams, the method of operation is quite different. Each team model provides a structure for team communication and interaction.

Multidisciplinary model

The multidisciplinary model was the first attempt to bring together professionals from a variety of disciplines to work as a team. Multidisciplinary team members work independently of one another. Peterson compares the mode of interaction among members of multidisciplinary teams to parallel play in young children—"side by side, but separate."[9(p484)] This comparison captures the spirit of many multidisciplinary teams. The work of each team member is viewed as important, but the team members are primarily concerned with the clinical issues of their own disciplines.

By design, practitioners on these teams operate more as independent specialists than as interactive team members.[2,7] Such independence can contribute to isolated and fragmented services for children and families.[3] Most often, families are not considered to be full members of the multidisciplinary team.

Multidisciplinary team members conduct separate assessments by discipline. Following the assessment, each team member generally writes a separate report, developing and implementing separate goals. Lack of coordination and communication among multidisciplinary team members places the responsibility for case management on the family.

Interdisciplinary model

The interdisciplinary model of team interaction was developed in response to many of the problems experienced by multidisciplinary teams. The interdisciplinary model builds on the strengths of the earlier model, but provides a formal structure for interaction and communication among team members that encourages the sharing of information.[2,9] Most often, the family is considered to be a member of the interdisciplinary team.

Interdisciplinary teams assess children and, sometimes families, independently by discipline. The team members come together to discuss their individual results and to plan cooperatively for intervention. Although the team develops a service plan jointly, each staff member is usually responsible for the part of the plan related to his or her professional disciplines. The plan is implemented by one person, often the educator, with scheduled therapy or consultation for the specialists on the team.

Problems in communication and interaction arise when interdisciplinary team members lack a full understanding of the professional training and expertise of the members from other disciplines on the team. Members may be confused about their role on the team, and their interaction may be complicated by issues of professional "turf."[2,8] As Howard states, many interdisciplinary teams have discovered that shared terminology does not always have shared meaning.[12]

Transdisciplinary model

The transdisciplinary model is an attempt to solve some of the problems of role confusion and team interaction that can result when team members from a variety of disciplines work together. The transdisciplinary team crosses disciplinary boundaries so that all team members teach and learn the basic terminology and simple intervention procedures of other disciplines represented on the team.[13] While there are differences in the degree of interaction among team members, the transdisciplinary model is similar in many ways to the interdisciplinary model.

One critical difference between the transdisciplinary approach and the other two models is the central role that families play on the transdisciplinary team. Although families may be part of the multidisciplinary team, and generally are part of the interdisciplinary team, they are full members of the transdisciplinary team. In fact, many transdisciplinary teams provide families with the option of serving as team captains, thus acknowledging their ultimate decision-making power.

The success of the transdisciplinary model depends on a process of formal and informal exchange that the United Cerebral Palsy's National Collaborative Infant Project calls "role release."[14] Role release is a conscious, carefully planned process that allows transdisciplinary team members to exchange information, knowledge, and skills across disciplines and to work as an integrated team.

All members of the transdisciplinary team assess the child together, using a format called the "arena assessment." During the arena assessment, all team members observe and record every aspect of the child's behavior during the arena. Only the family and one other team member, who serves as the assessment facilitator, interact with and handle the child, a factor that reduces the potentially disruptive effect of having many persons present at the arena. While there have been few comparative studies conducted so far, one, by Woolery and Dyk, reports that both parents and professionals have judged the arena assessment to be more beneficial than individual and isolated assessments by each discipline.[15]

The entire transdisciplinary team also develops an integrated service plan and authorizes ones person, usually called the "primary service provider" or "case manager," to carry out the plan with the family. All team members share equal responsibility for the success of the plan by providing formal and informal support to the family and the primary service provider. When complicated interventions require specific disciplinary expertise, backup support and therapy are provided by the team member from the appropriate discipline.

THE FAMILY AS TEAM MEMBER

Regardless of the team interaction model chosen by individual programs, Public Law 99-457 clearly directs teams to work together with the family to plan for and provide early intervention services to infants and toddlers with special needs. The requirement that infants and toddlers be provided services in a family context represents an evolution of the family's role in early intervention.

Turnbull and Summers[16] have traced the history of this evolution from an early view of parents as part of the problem to a more recent emphasis on parent "involvement"—the idea that parents should be intervenors or cotherapists with their children. Parent involvement or participation has been a dominant theme in early intervention for more than ten years.

In recognition of the primary influence that families have on their child's development, the best practice until very recently directed early interventionists to involve parents at all costs. This effort typically took the form of obtaining parental approval of program plans, training parents to carry out these plans at home, and providing opportunities for counseling or participation in parent groups. Parents were encouraged to be team members, but their role on the team often was limited to rubber-stamping the recommendations of the professional team members.

The importance of parental participation and involvement was a belief so firmly held that many early intervention programs would not serve children whose parents were unable or unwilling to participate in the program. The goal of these programs was to help children by helping families—to share their information and experience as professionals so that parents could help their children as much as possible.

The flaw in this approach was in the interpretation of "helping" families. Many programs were directive in their interactions with families, firmly believing in the wisdom of their recommendations for children and, by extension, for families. Goals for the child or family were often not shared by the family and, sometimes, were not even consistent with the family's priorities or values. Turnbull and Turnbull[17] and Bailey[18] have documented the frequent incongruence between the family's and professional's priorities and insights.

When families inevitably failed to become involved in programs as expected—participating in program planning meetings, coming to parent groups, or carrying out program plans at home—professionals sometimes became frustrated or angry, labeling such parents as "difficult" or "noncompliant." Parents, in turn, were frustrated with early intervention services that were intrusive, directive, or unrealistic. Turnbull and Summers, reflecting on the demands that many early intervention staff place on parents' time at home, write that "anything is possible to those with no responsibility for implementation."[16(p10)]

As the field of early intervention has matured, however, many parents and professionals alike have come to regard the concept of parental involvement as counterproductive. The early intervention literature recently took a new look at the philosophies and practices relating to families and offered an enabling and empowering approach that recognizes and builds on the strengths and resources present in all families.[11,19–24]

Best practice is shifting from an emphasis on parental involvement or participation to an emphasis on family-focused services. Families are being viewed as competent decision makers who must be allowed to choose their level of involvement with an early intervention program according to their values, resources, strengths, needs, and supports.

Dunst[19] writes that, while early intervention practitioners may always have sensed these ideas to be true, they lacked in the past a conceptual framework to enable them to act on their intuition. Systems theories provide this framework for a family-focused approach to early intervention.[19,25,26]

A family-focused approach requires that early intervention practitioners redefine the family's role on the team and, perhaps, early intervention itself. Dunst and associates[21] define early intervention in a new way that recognizes the strengths of families and encourages a new professional role. Early intervention, then, is "the provision of support (i.e., resources provided by others) by members of a family's informal and formal social network that either directly or indirectly influences child, parent, and family functioning."[21(p7)]

If widely accepted and put into practice, this new view of early intervention as the provision of support to further strengthen, enable, and empower families may change the entire character of the field. The first step for professionals is to recognize behaviors that operate against this enabling principle. Bailey describes common helping behavior by early intervention practitioners as follows:

> we often find that when a problem is mentioned by parents, early interventionists are eager to offer solutions or services to solve the problem. Interventionists view this as a positive professional characteristic since they are responding to parents' needs. Furthermore, it is self-reinforcing and an exercise of power to be able to dispense solutions to families.[18(p64)]

As early intervention professionals seek new ways to interact with families, they must develop new roles and incorporate them into their professional identities. Dunst et al[21] have identified eight nonmutually exclusive roles for early intervention staff: empathetic listener, teacher-therapist, consultant, resource, enabler, mobilizer, mediator, and advocate. Among the activities associated with these roles are "linking people, mobilizing existing resources and support, facilitating the establishment of new support structures, moderating exchanges among network members, (and) consulting with families about problems or concerns."[27(p28)]

Although some of these roles and activities are very familiar to early interventionists, others will require a substantial change in perspective and behavior. The development and implementation of IFSPs provide a unique, timely opportunity for practitioners to make such changes.

THE INDIVIDUALIZED FAMILY SERVICE PLAN

The IFSP, if approached from a family systems perspective, may be a radical change for many early intervention programs. Most practitioners have been developing service plans based on the "IEP model." Whether these plans were called individualized development, habilitation, education, or service plans, they typically were formulated by program staff based on assessment data on the child's developmental status, with varying degrees of family participation in the process.

Although many programs did include "family" goals in their service plans, these goals often were based on the *staff's perceptions* of the family's needs. Goals were frequently written in terms of family compliance with the program's priorities and procedures. The mandated IFSP challenges early intervention teams to develop instruments and practices that allow families to assess their own needs and that encourage collaborative IFSP goal setting.

Public Law 99-457 specifies the content of the IFSP, as well as certain participation requirements and implementation procedures. Part H, section 677, requires that the IFSP be developed by a team made up of professionals from multiple disciplines and the parent or guardian. The IFSP must be in writing and must contain:

- a statement of the child's present levels of physical development, cognitive development, language and speech development, psychosocial development, and self-help skills, based on acceptable, objective criteria;
- a statement of the family's strengths and needs related to enhancing the development of the family's handicapped infant or toddler;
- a statement of the major outcomes expected to be achieved for the child and family; the criteria, procedures, and time lines used to determine the degree to which progress is being made; and whether or not revisions of the outcomes or services are necessary;
- a statement of specific early intervention services necessary to meet the unique needs of the child and family, including the frequency, intensity, and method of delivering services;
- the projected dates for the initiation of services and the anticipated duration of the services;
- the name of case manager (from the profession most immediately relevant to the child's or family's needs) who will be responsible for implementing the plan and coordinating with other agencies and persons; and
- the steps to be taken supporting the child's transition to part B preschool services, to the extent that such services are appropriate.

Some of the above provisions are already being addressed in service plans in programs across the country, while others are new. Many practitioners are confused about what the new requirements mean. How should they assess the family's needs? How will they decide what services programs and agencies should offer families? What should a team do when families identify needs that their program is not able to meet? What happens when the staff and family disagree on priorities for services?

Assessing the family's needs

Assessing the family's needs is a special challenge for early intervention practitioners, many of whom have little or no training in family systems or family-centered approaches to services. Bailey and Simeonsson[28] have provided a helpful discussion of the complicated issues surrounding the assessment of the family's needs in early intervention. Traditionally, psychologists and social workers have accepted the responsibility for family assessment. Program staff from these disciplines were trained to evaluate the family's needs in a number of dimensions, using instruments that frequently focused on deficits, assumed psychopathology, or required sophisticated interpretation and inferential reasoning.[28]

In general, other early intervention team members have had little experience in assessing the family's needs. Now that such assessment is a required part of the IFSP, programs need instruments that can be used by all team members. The instruments should reflect the program's respect for the family's ability to make its own decisions.

Procedures to assess the family's needs must also provide "systematic and multiple opportunities" for families to express their needs and concerns in both open-ended and structured formats.[18(p67)] In addition, family assessment instruments and practices must be flexible because of the diversity of families. As Chandler et al note, "families may vary in their structure, ethnic and cultural backgrounds, economic status, educational resources, ideologies, personal and mental health problems, and coping styles for dealing with problems."[29(p234)]

Many exemplary early intervention programs are choosing a variety of family needs assessments that stress self-reporting on the part of the family. Only when families have the opportunity to identify their own needs and priorities can service plans accurately reflect family goals.

The Family, Infant and Preschool Program (FIPP) in Morganton, NC, has developed a number of family needs assessments from a family enabling perspective. The FIPP provides both home- and center-based early intervention services to approximately 300 families. The needs-based assessment and intervention strategy at FIPP involves the identification of the family's needs and sources of support and resources to meet those needs and specifies staff roles in helping families find and use the resources in their support network.

Among the family assessments developed and used at FIPP are the Family Support Scale, the Family Resource Scale, the Support Functions Scale, and the Family Needs Scale. All of these instruments involve self-reporting by the family. Using information gathered from these and other assessments, FIPP staff and families develop a "map" of the families' social support network that can be used to develop family service plans. Dunst et al have published data on the reliability, validity, and other characteristics of these instruments, as well as a description of the various scales.[21,30]

Child Development Resources (CDR), a private nonprofit agency in Lightfoot, Va, provides early intervention services to infants and toddlers with special needs and their families. CDR uses a team-based assessment process that allows the family to determine their own service needs. The staff members function as consultants to the family, helping them to identify needs of the child and family and discussing the menu of service options. Once families have decided on their service needs, they work with other team members to identify their own strengths and resources relative to meeting those needs.

Families are not asked to provide information that does not directly address the already identified needs, thus reducing the intrusiveness of the information gathering. Families are provided continuing opportunities to identify their needs so that they feel free to choose how much information they want to share or reveal at any given time.

The Family Needs Survey developed by Bailey and Simeonsson at the Frank Porter Graham Center of the University of North Carolina at Chapel Hill is one instrument that gives families an opportunity to tell staff directly what their needs are in six areas: information, support, explanations to others, community services, finances, and family functioning. The instrument consists of 35 statements relating to common needs of families in these six areas. A simple rating scale allows families to clearly state their needs.[28]

Developing IFSP goals

After the family's needs have been assessed, the next step is translating those needs into goals for the IFSP. This is a difficult step for many programs because it requires negotiation, collaboration, and mutual problem solving between the professional members of the team and the family.[18]

It is at this point in the early intervention process that family and staff differences in perspective, values, and priorities most often surface. Practitioners traditionally have focused on the therapeutic and educational needs of the child, often to the exclusion of other family considerations. Perhaps the most controversial aspect of a family systems, enabling approach to early intervention is the principle that, when family and staff perceptions of need differ, the service goals reflect the priorities and values of the family rather than those of the staff.

This principle of family direction does not devalue the perspective and skills of early intervention practitioners.[18] Rather, it recognizes that "a person's perception of what constitutes the most important needs at a particular time will likely assume priority status and guide the person's behavior."[23(p249)]

Acknowledging this principle frees early intervention practitioners from the frustration of developing goals and service plans that are meaningful only when staff members are actually working directly with the child. The challenge for professionals is to learn new ways to negotiate collaborative goals with families that allow practitioners to share their information, skills, and recommendations in a way that supports rather than supplants the family's role.

Bailey lists five basic skills that early intervention staff need to develop goals collaboratively with families: "the ability to (1) view a family from a systems perspective; (2) systematically assess relevant family needs; (3) use effective listening and interviewing techniques; (4) negotiate values and priorities to reach a joint solution; and (5) act as 'case managers' in helping families match needs with available community resources."[18(p64)]

Public Law 99-457 does not state or imply that the IFSP must contain goals that address all of a family's needs. Rather, in section 677 teams are directed to consider the family's strengths and needs related to enhancing the development of their child. This is a critical distinction. It is beyond the scope of most early intervention programs to meet all of the needs of all families. Clearly, some problems are beyond the skills and resources available in many programs. Among these, according to Bailey, are "serious marital discord, unemployment, financial impoverishment, chronic personality problems, and limited parent cognitive abilities."[18(p69)]

When such problems are present and when the family perceives them to be problems, the staff and family can work together to determine desired outcomes and can identify supports and resources in the community. It is particularly important that needs be perceived by the family, rather than by the staff alone. Staff team members should avoid making judgments about family relationships based on their own values. Making such judgments frequently results in a hidden agenda—unacknowledged staff goals for changes in the family.

As teams begin to develop goals, a natural inclination is to turn to their experience in developing goals for the child—the IEP model discussed earlier. Unfortunately, this model does not lend itself readily to developing goals for the family. After years of practice in writing behavioral objectives for children with measurable criteria for child change, early intervention practitioners must redirect their thinking. While teachers set goals for change in children's behavior and are responsible for bringing about this change, early interventionists have a different role and relationship in working with families.

Early interventionists can provide families with the information and support that enables them to direct their own strengths and resources to bring about their desired outcomes. The goal of this type of help is not a behavioral change in the family in the same sense that the goal of therapy with a child is a behavioral change in the child, such as better head control or the elimination of head banging.

If practitioners do not recognize this difference, they are likely to impose goals on the family that are directive, judgmental, or paternalistic, or that meet the needs of the program rather than those of the family. The following is an example of a "family" goal developed by staff in one program who forgot this important distinction: "When the home visitor arrives at the home, Mrs Smith will be up and dressed and will have Travis dressed and fed at least 90% of the time." The staff measured the progress toward meeting this objective by counting the number of times Mrs Smith took more than five minutes after the home visitor arrived to get herself and her son ready for the visit.

Such a goal clearly is not consistent with an enabling and empowering approach to families. Yet, because it was directed at the mother rather than the child, the staff considered it a family goal. If practitioners are to make the most of the IFSP, they must guard against the temptation to use family goals as a means to increase family compliance with program policies and procedures.

• • •

In light of Public Law 99-457, early intervention programs are facing new challenges. The IFSP requirement of part H challenges practitioners to choose new models for team interaction and to develop the skills needed to work in true, collaborative partnerships with families. The current movement toward a family systems, family-centered approach to early intervention suggests that the most appropriate team models are those that are highly interactive and that consider the family to be a full member of the team—in fact, the team member with the final decision-making power.

Many families have expressed concern that a family-focused approach to early intervention may result in yet one more professional expectation of proper family behavior. These families fear that program staff will interpret the new approach to mean that all families should act as their own case managers, make decisions alone, or be active and involved in all aspects of an early intervention program.

A family-focused approach encourages just the opposite. Far from prescribing a required role for all families, family-centered programs give families many options, including the opportunity to choose the level of team participation that is most comfortable for them at any given time. Some families will take a leadership role, choosing assessment instruments and procedures, developing IFSP goals that the rest of the team will help implement, and selecting program services that best match their child's needs. Other families, at least initially, will opt for a different level of interaction and involvement with a program, expecting the staff to take the leading role in programming decisions.

When programs and professionals provide families with the opportunity to make conscious and informed choices from an array of options, they ensure that a family's association with early intervention truly meets family needs, rather than meeting program needs, expectations, and demands. Now that Public Law 99-457 is a reality, early intervention practitioners are asking how to best make a place for families on their early intervention teams.

A more appropriate question might be posed such as how early intervention professionals can become part of the family's team, on which the family already functions as team captain and decisionmaker. Professionals can offer help in response to expressed needs and offer support that enables families to draw from their own resources to enhance the development of their children with special needs.

REFERENCES

1. Gilkerson L, Hillard AG, Schrag E, et al: *Report Accompanying the Education of the Handicapped Act Amendments (Report #99-860) and Comments on P.L. 99-457.* Washington, DC, National Maternal and Child Health Clearinghouse, 1987.
2. Fewell RR: The team approach to infant education, in Garwood SG, Fewell RR (eds): *Educating Handicapped Infants: Issues in Development and Intervention.* Rockville, Md, Aspen Publishers, 1983.
3. Woodruff G, McGonigel MJ: Early intervention team models: The transdisciplinary approach, in Gallagher JJ, Hutinger P, Jordan JB, et al (eds): *Early Childhood Special Education: Birth to Three.* Reston, Va, Council for Exceptional Children, in press.
4. Woodruff G, McGonigel MJ, Garland CW, et al: *Planning Programs for Infants,* TADS State Series Paper No. 2. Chapel Hill, NC, University of North Carolina at Chapel Hill, 1985.
5. Holm VA, McCartin RE: Interdisciplinary child development team: Team issues and training in interdisciplinariness, in Allen KE, Holm VA, Schiefelbusch RL (eds): *Early Intervention—A Team Approach.* Baltimore, Md, University Park Press, 1978.
6. Dyer WG: *Team Building: Issues and Alternatives.* Reading, Mass, Addison-Wesley, 1977.
7. Bennett FC: The pediatrician and the interdisciplinary process. *Except Child* 1982;48:306–314.
8. Linder T: *Early Childhood Special Education: Program Development and Administration.* Baltimore, Md, Brookes, 1983.
9. Peterson N: *Early Intervention for Handicapped and At-Risk Children: An Introduction to Early Childhood Special Education.* Denver, Colo, Love, 1987.
10. Bailey DB: A triaxial model of the interdisciplinary team and group process. *Except Child* 1984;51:17–25.
11. Healy A, Keesee PD, Smith BS: *Early Services for Children With Special Needs: Transactions for Family Support.* Iowa City, Iowa, University of Iowa, 1985.
12. Howard J: The role of the pediatrician with young exceptional children and their families. *Except Child.* 1982;48:316–322.
13. Haynes U: The National Collaborative Infant Project, in Tjossem TD (ed): *Intervention Strategies for High Risk Infants and Young Children.* Baltimore, Md. University Park Press, 1976.
14. United Cerebral Palsy National Collaborative Infant Project: *Staff Development Handbook: A Resource for the Transdisciplinary Process.* New York, United Cerebral Palsy Associations of America, 1976.
15. Woolery M, Dyk L: Arena assessment: Description and preliminary social validity data. *J Assoc Persons Severe Handicaps* 1984;9:231–235.
16. Turnbull AP, Summers JA: From family involvement to family support: Evolution to revolution. Presented at the Down's Syndrome State-of-the-Art Conference, Boston, Mass, April 24, 1985.
17. Turnbull AP, Turnbull HR: *Parents Speak Out: Then and Now.* Columbus, Ohio, Charles E. Merrill, 1985.

18. Bailey DB: Collaborative goal setting with families: Resolving differences in values and priorities for services. *Top Early Child Spec Educ* 1987;7(2):59–71.
19. Dunst CJ: Emerging trends and advances in early intervention programs. *NJ J Sch Psychol* 1983;2:26–40.
20. Dunst CJ, Trivette CM: Enabling and empowering families: Conceptual and intervention issues. *Sch Psychol Rev* 1987;16:443–456.
21. Dunst CJ, Trivette CM, Deal AG: *Enabling and Empowering Families.* Cambridge, Mass, Brookline, in press.
22. Hobbs N, Dokecki PR, Hoover-Dempsey KV, et al: *Strengthening Families: Strategies for Improved Child Care and Parent Education.* San Francisco, Jossey-Bass, 1984.
23. Trivette CM, Deal A, Dunst CJ: Family needs, sources of support, and professional roles: Critical elements of family systems assessment and intervention. *Diagnostique* 1986;11:246–267.
24. Turnbull AP, Turnbull HR: *Families, Professionals, and Exceptionalities: A Special Partnership.* Columbus, Ohio, Charles E. Merrill, 1986.
25. Bronfenbrenner U: *The Ecology of Human Development: Experiments by Nature and Design.* Cambridge, Mass, Harvard University Press, 1979.
26. Foster M, Berger M, McLean M: Rethinking a good idea: A reassessment of parent involvement. *Top Early Child Spec Educ* 1981;1(3):55–65.
27. Dunst CJ, Leet HE, Trivette C: Family resources, personal well-being, and early intervention. *J Spec Educ,* in press.
28. Bailey DB, Simeonsson RJ: Assessing needs of families with handicapped infants: The Family Needs Survey. *Top Early Child Spec Educ,* in press.
29. Chandler LK, Fowler SA, Lubeck RC: Assessing family needs: The first step in providing family focused intervention. *Diagnostique* 1986;11:233–245.
30. Dunst CJ, Jenkins V, Trivette CM: The family support scale: Reliability and validity. *J Individ Fam Community Wellness* 1984;1(4):45–52.

Index

Page numbers in *italics* denote figures; those followed by "T" denote tables.

I

K

L

M